Assessing Community Health Programs

A Trainer's Guide

Using LQAS for Baseline Surveys and Regular Monitoring

Joseph J. Valadez, PhD, MPH, ScD
William Weiss, MA
Corey Leburg, MHS
Robb Davis, PhD, MPH

Teaching-aids At Low Cost (TALC), St Albans (UK)
Illustrations by The Hesperian Foundation

Published by:
Teaching-aids At Low Cost.
PO Box 49 St Albans Herts AL1 5TX UK

www.talcuk.org

ISBN: 0-9544894-0-3

All rights reserved.

First Published 2003
Text © Joseph J. Valadez
Illustrations © Hesperian Foundation

TALC (Teaching-aids At Low Cost) is a UK registered charity (no: 279858) and a Company limited by guarantee registered in England (no: 1477636) which supplies teaching-aids and books to raise standards of health care and reduce poverty worldwide.

Although every effort has been made to ensure the completeness and accuracy of the information contained in this publication, TALC cannot be held responsible for any recommendations contained therein or any errors that may have inadvertently occurred. TALC shall not, therefore, be liable under any circumstances whatsoever, for any damages suffered as a result of any such errors, omissions or recommendations arising from the use of this publication.

Cover design: Hesperian Foundation

Graphics and Design: Hesperian Foundation

Copy Editing: Freedom From Hunger

Structure, Training and Typesetting: Valadez, Weiss, Leburg, and Davis

Printed by: Photolit Printing Ltd. [St Albans. England]

We dedicate this book to community health workers and local program supervisors working to improve the health of people in communities throughout the world. We also dedicate this book to our mothers—special people in our lives.

Copyright © 2003 by Joseph J. Valadez. All rights reserved.
First Printing January 2003

NGOs, PVOs, International Organizations, Ministries of Health, universities may reproduce these materials for educational purposes or to improve health programs. None of these materials may be reproduced for commercial purposes without written permission.

This publication was made possible through support provided by the Bureau for Global Health, U.S. Agency for International Development, under the terms of Award No. HRN-A-00-98-00011-00. The opinions expressed herein are those of the authors and do not necessarily reflect the views of the U.S. Agency for International Development.

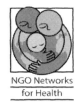
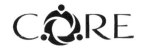

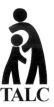

Teaching-aids At Low Cost (TALC)
PO Box 49
St Albans, Herts
AL1 5TX UK
Tel: 00 44 (0) 1727 853869
Fax: 00 44 (0) 1727 846852
Email: info@talcuk.org
Website: www.talcuk.org

TABLE OF CONTENTS

A Trainer's Guide: Using LQAS for Baseline Surveys and Regular Monitoring

Acknowledgements — Page vi

Introduction — Page viii

MODULE ONE: Why should I do a survey and why should I use the LQAS method? — Page 1

Session 1: Introducing Participants and the Training/Survey — page 2

> Overhead #1—Getting to Know One Another
> Overhead #2—Purpose of the LQAS Workshop
> Overhead #3—Skills To Be Learned
> Overhead #4—Overview of the LQAS Training Program
> Overhead #5—Abbreviated Training Schedule/Agenda
> Overhead #6—Defining Catchment Area and Supervision Areas

Session 2: Uses of Surveys — page 7

> Overhead #7—What Is Coverage?
> Overhead #8—What Surveys Can Show You
> Overhead #9—NGO Program Area: Scenario 1
> Overhead #10—NGO Program Area: Scenario 2
> Overhead #11—NGO Program Area: Scenario 3
> Overhead #12—Using Survey Data
> Overhead #13—Uses of Surveys

Session 3: Random Sampling — page 13

> Overhead #14—Why Sample?

Session 4: Using LQAS Sampling for Surveys — page 20

> Overhead #15—NGO Program Area: Scenario 4
> Overhead #16—LQAS Sampling Results
> Overhead #17—The LQAS Table
> Overhead #18—What a Sample of 19 Can Tell Us
> Overhead #19—What a Sample of 19 Cannot Tell Us
> Overhead #20—Why Use a Sample of 19?

Session 5: Using LQAS for Baseline Surveys page 29

> Overhead #21—Five Supervision Areas and One Indicator
> Overhead #22—LQAS Concepts for Baseline Surveys
> Overhead #23—Five Supervision Areas and One Indicator: Participant Worksheet
> Overhead #24—Supervision Area A and Five Indicators
> Overhead #25—Comparing Supervision Areas A, B, C, D, and E

MODULE TWO: Where should I conduct my survey? page 38

Session 1: Identifying Interview Locations page 39

> Overhead #1—Identifying Locations for Interviews
> Overhead #2—List of Communities and Total Population for a Supervision Area
> Overhead #3—Calculate the Cumulative Population
> Overhead #4—Calculate the Sampling Interval
> Overhead #5—Random Number Table
> Overhead #6—Identify the Location of Each of the 19 Interviews in a Supervision Area: Worksheet
> Overhead #7—LQAS Sampling Frame for a Supervision Area

MODULE THREE: Whom should I interview? page 49

Session 1: Selecting Households page 50

> Overhead #1—How To Assign Numbers to Households
> Overhead #2—Situation 2: Household List Not Available—Size About 30
> Overhead #3—Situation 3: Household List Not Available—Size Greater Than 30
> Overhead #4—Group of 27 Households Numbered for Random Selection of 1 Household

Session 2: Selecting Respondents page 56

> Overhead #5— Rules for Identifying Respondents
> Overhead #6— Household Composition Scenarios

Session 3: Field Practical for Numbering and Selecting Households page 60

> Overhead #7—Process for Field Practical

MODULE FOUR: What questions do I ask and how should I ask them?   **Page 66**

Session 1: Reviewing the Survey Questionnaires   page 67

> No overheads

Session 2: Interviewing Skills   page 69

> Overhead #1—Why Interviewing is Important
> Overhead #2—Interview Etiquette
> Overhead #3—Effective Interviewing Techniques

Session 3: Field Practical for Interviewing   page 73

> No overheads

Session 4: Planning and Doing the Data Collection/Survey   page 76

> HANDOUT - Survey Checklists

MODULE FIVE: What do I do with the information I have collected during the baseline survey?   **Page 78**

Session 1: Fieldwork Debriefing   page 79

> Overhead #1—Status Report on Data Collection from the NGO

Session 2: Tabulating Results   page 81

> Overhead #2— Result Tabulation Table
> HANDOUT—Tabulation Quality Checklist

Session 3: Analyzing Results   page 89

> Overhead #3—Summary Tabulation Sheet for Baseline Surveys
> Overhead #4—The LQAS Table
> Overhead #5—Defining Program Goals and Annual Targets
> Overhead #6—Monitoring Targets and Average Coverage Over Time: In a Catchment Area
> Overhead #7—How To Analyze Data and Identify Priorities Using the Summary Tables
> Overhead #8—Baseline Survey Report Format
> Overhead #9—Methodology
> Overhead #10—Main Findings
> Overhead #11—Action Plans/Goals/Coverage Targets for Key Indicators

MODULE SIX: What do I do with the information I have collected during regular monitoring? Page 95

Session 1: Fieldwork Debriefing page 96

> Overhead #1—Status Report on Data Collettion from the NGO

Session 2: Tabulating Results page 98

> Overhead #2—Result Tabulation Table
> HANDOUT—Tabulation Quality Checklist

Session 3: Analyzing Results page 106

> Overhead #3—Summary Tabulation Sheet for Regular Monitoring
> Overhead #4—The LQAS Table
> Overhead #5—Defining Program Goals and Annual Targets
> Overhead #6—How to Identify Priority SAs Using the Summary Tables During Regular Monitoring
> Overhead #7—Using LQAS to Assess One Indicator Over the Life of a Project
> Overhead #8—Monitoring Targets and Average Coverage Over Time: In a Catchment Area
> Overhead #9—How To Analyze Data and Identify Priorities Using the Summary Tables
> Overhead #10—Monitoring Survey Report Format
> Overhead #11—Methodology
> Overhead #12—Main Findings
> Overhead #13—Action Plans/Goals/Coverage Targets for Key Indicators

APPENDICES		page A-1
Appendix 1:	Sample Workshop Agenda	Page A-2
Appendix 2:	Dealing with More Than One Respondent Type—Parallel Sampling - Identifying Interviewees - Interviewing Subgroups of Interviewees - Parallel Sampling and Developing a Questionnaire - How to Parallel Sample	Page A-9
Appendix 3:	LQAS Table with Alpha and Beta Errors n=19 - What Is an Alpha and Beta Error? - Why Use a Sample of 19?	Page A-13
Appendix 4:	Additional Random Number Tables	Page A-16
Appendix 5:	Alternative Neighborhood/Community Scenarios	Page A-19
Appendix 6:	How to Calculate Weighted Coverage and Confidence Intervals - Calculating Weighted Coverage Proportions With a Confidence Interval by Hand - Calculating Weighted Coverage Proportions with a Confidence Interval with a Computer - How Many SAs Should I Have?	Page A-23
Appendix 7:	Example Tabulation Tables for Sub-Samples in which You Use Aggregate Measures Only - Results Table Exclusive Breastfeeding - Results Table Diarrhea Prevalence and Case Management - Summary Table Exclusive Breastfeeding - Summary Table Diarrhea Prevalence and Case Management	Page A-29

PART II   A Participant's Manual and Workbook: Using LQAS for Baseline Surveys and Regular Monitoring   Page PM-1

IMPORTANT: Each overhead cited in the trainer's guide appears as a handout in the Participant's Manual and Workbook (which is simply a collection of these overheads). While the trainer works from the overhead, participants can follow along on their Manual/Workbook.

Acknowledgments:

The authors would like to thank all those in the field who have helped us to create this guide. Your feedback during various field tests has improved this product, and your patience and understanding made working with you a great pleasure. We hope you will take well-deserved satisfaction from knowing the important part you played in making this valuable tool available to your colleagues and friends around the world. In particular we would like to thank several networks of non-governmental organizations working in Nicaragua, Malawi and Armenia who participated in using earlier versions of this guide and in making many useful suggestions about how to improve it. They include:

NICASALUD whose members include:
- ADP
- ADRA
- ALISTAR
- CARE
- Catholic Relief Services
- CEPS
- Compañeros
- FUNDEMUNI
- INPRHU
- IXCHEN
- Hablemos
- Partners of the Americas
- Plan International
- Project Concern International
- Project Hope
- Save the Children

UMOYO NETWORKS, whose members include:
- Adventist Health Services
- Word Alive Ministries International
- Ekwendeni Hospital
- MACRO
- Malamolo Hospital

ARMENIA NETWORK FOR HEALTH, whose members include:
- ADRA
- CARE
- Save the Children

Special recognition is given to Babu Ram Devkota of Plan International, Nepal and his team working in the Child Survival Project in the Terai. Babu Ram, Eric Starbuck, and the Plan Program Supervisors tested most of the methods presented here. We also give our deep thanks to William Vargas of Costa Rica, who used draft versions of this guide in Central and South America and in Malawi. Without his help and dedication this guide would not have been possible.

In the USA we thank Dr. Peter Winch, Dr. Eric Sarriot and other members of the faculty of the Department of International Health at the Johns Hopkins University Bloomberg School of Public Health. Their recent review article of sampling methods is an important contribution to Public Health. It has also created awareness among PVOs and NGOs that LQAS, as well as other sampling approaches, are important tools for improving the quality of community health programs. Among our donors we would like to thank Kate Jones and the staff of the Bureau of Humanitarian Relief's Office of Private Voluntary Cooperation at USAID. Craig Storti provided a great service to us as our editor, Brenda Bolanos helped the authors format the guide to make it more user-friendly and La Rue Seims copied the decision rules from earlier LQAS tables into the one used in the article. Warm thanks to Freedom from Hunger who edited the manual. Thanks also to the Hesperian Foundation and Gayton Design for production assistance.

In conclusion, we express our gratitude to the many public health professionals who have been advancing the development of LQAS throughout Asia, Africa, and Central and South America as well as to the members of the Child Survival Collaborations and Resources Group (CORE) for their support and interest which provided the impetus to develop this guide. Many PVO members of CORE field tested this Guide and the Manual/Workbook. Their comments helped to improve them. Without the support of the NGO Networks for Health Project it would not have been possible to develop the Trainer's Guide and Participant's Manual and Workbook.

INTRODUCTION

This guide is for managers, field supervisors, and others who plan, monitor and evaluate community health programs. Most often, the people who have such a responsibility also have to collect data as one of their tasks. The guide will aid them to train others in a simple and rapid method for collecting data to use for planning, monitoring and evaluating community health programs. The method is called Lot Quality Assurance Sampling (LQAS). LQAS has been used by industry for about 75 years for quality-control purposes. But it has been adapted for use by community health practitioners over the past 15 years. LQAS is now used all over the world in community health programs for the following purposes: (1) assessing coverage of key health knowledge and practices in maternal and child health, family planning, and HIV/AIDS; (2) assessing the quality of health worker performance; and (3) assessing disease prevalence. This guide presents LQAS in a very user-friendly way so that almost any supervisor or community health worker can be trained in how to use the method for the first purpose mentioned above—which is the most often-used application.

This guide is written from the view of NGOs as the users. However, all the materials can be easily adapted for any other user. We encourage Ministry of Health staff, UN Agencies and any others to use this guide. Whereever you read NGO or NGO catchment area, think of a large area that corresponds to your administrative unit. For example, an NGO catchment area could be a district or sub-district area.

The guide consists of two sections: (1) a guide for trainers—for anyone, that is, who wants or needs to train other people in the LQAS methodology; and (2) a participant's manual or workbook, which is simply a collection of all the overheads/handouts used in the training program.

The guide consists of six Modules, each with one or more separate Sessions, with each Module answering a key question about data collection. These questions are:

> MODULE ONE: Why should I do a survey and why should I use the LQAS method?
>
> MODULE TWO: Where should I conduct my survey?
>
> MODULE THREE: Whom should I interview?

MODULE FOUR:	What questions do I ask and how should I ask them?
MODULE FIVE:	What do I do with the information I have collected during the baseline survey?
MODULE SIX:	What do I do with the information I have collected during regular monitoring?

Each Session has the same layout:

PURPOSE The Session begins with a brief purpose statement which tells the trainer why he or she is doing this Session and where the Session fits in with the overall design of the training program. Trainers might also want to use some of the comments here when they introduce this Session to participants.

TIME This tells the trainer about how long it should take to complete this Session. Times will vary, of course, depending on the number and experience of participants, among other things.

OBJECTIVES This section describes what participants will achieve in this Session.

PREPARATION This describes for trainers anything they need to do before the Session.

DELIVERY This section leads trainers step-by-step through the entire Session and explains what they should do and say at each point in the Session.

GRAPHICS This symbol signals when the trainer should display an overhead. The number (#) is the overhead number for the module being discussed. This number corresponds to the numbered overhead in the Participant's Manual and Workbook.

Introduction

> IMPORTANT: The most important thing for trainers is to be completely familiar with every step in every Session, including all the overheads, <u>before they stand up in front of the group</u>. Trainers should not be trying to figure out the Session at the same time they are delivering it!

A list of all the modules, Sessions and Session overheads/handouts appears in the Table of Contents.

How to Prepare for the Training

Before the training begins, there are several things that need to be prepared for the workshop Modules to be successful. Go through the following list and carry out these tasks well before the workshop.

TASK 1—Get a map of the catchment area where the NGO will collect the data.
This can be a formal map on which the NGO has clearly marked the boundaries of their program area—the catchment area. Try to find a map that gives you maximum detail and has a small scale. It is even better if it has roads, community names, and geographical characteristics marked on it. You can often find maps at the Department of Statistics or the Census. If the Demographic and Health Survey has been conducted in your country, there are often maps available to use locally. Other sources of maps are tourist agencies, military institutes, and the Departments of Health and Education. School Districts often have maps. But if a map is not available, then ask the NGO to sketch one by hand. It will be useful for the training and for carrying out the survey.

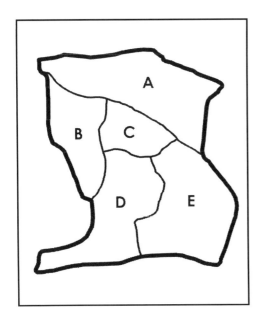

TASK 2—Work with NGO managers to decide how to organize their program area or catchment area into supervision areas.
During this training we will use the phrase *supervision area* many times. Sometimes we will abbreviate it as SA. An NGO can make program monitoring and supervision much easier if they subdivide their program catchment area into smaller management units. As shown in the figure to the left, together, A, B, C, D, and E represent the **Catchment Area**. Individually, A, B, C, D, and E represent five **Supervision Areas**.

A. Each management unit is called a supervision area. The data you get will be strongest—meeting accepted international standards—if you subdivide the program area into at least five SAs. But do not worry if for your program you can only divide into four SAs. But do try to have at least three SAs.

> **HINT: It will be much easier to use the list of communities later on if the NGO also indicates the district or province.**

B. The easiest way for an NGO to organize a program into SAs is to think about how many communities a supervisor can supervise in a month or 6 weeks. Then group communities that are a natural grouping and that make supervision the most efficient. Those communities form your supervision area. Because monitoring should be carried out regularly by a supervisor, and because this guide will teach supervisors how to collect data, encourage the NGO to define an SA that a supervisor can effectively manage. Once the NGO has done this, be sure they have identified supervisors who will do this work and will be committed to visiting the communities in that SA.

TASK 3—Develop a list of all the communities in the program area with their population sizes.

A. Ask the NGO to make a list in one column of all the communities in their program area, organized by SA. In a second column ask them to write the estimated population size of each one. If they do not know how many people live in each one, they can write down the estimated number of houses or the numbers of babies that were born in each one. Health facilities may have this information. The NGOs will need some information that helps them decide the relative size of each community. Don't worry too much if the estimates are not exact.

B. In Module 3, participants will learn how to use the list of communities as a sampling frame to identify interview locations. The trainer should work with one program manager at the NGO to identify the communities where the sampling will take place. In other words, go to Module 3 now and apply the steps described to identify locations. Later in the training you can lead participants through this process and show how the actual sampling frame was developed.

TASK 4—Prepare the questionnaires.
This may seem like an obvious task, but it is time-consuming and complex. You only learn how complex it is by actually developing the questionnaire.

A. Have the NGO write a list with each of the program's objectives related to improving health knowledge or practices. Under each objective, have the NGO write the key health message the project will promote to help achieve the objective. Under each objective, have the NGO write an indicator that can measure whether or not the objective has been achieved. The numerator and denominator of each indicator should be very specific as to gender and age group, and what is considered "correct" knowledge or practice.

   Here is an example: Let's assume that a project objective is that within four years 70 percent of women will know at least 3 ways to prevent HIV transmission. The indicator for this objective is the percentage of women who know at least three ways to prevent HIV transmission. The numerator is the total number of women interviewed in the survey whose responses show that they know at least 3 acceptable ways to prevent HIV transmission. The denominator is the number of women interviewed in the survey.

B. Have the NGO look for and select questions needed to measure each of the indicators written in the step above. The NGO can sometimes find the questions it needs by looking at a questionnaire that has already been used either by the NGO or by a colleague NGO. If the NGO cannot find a questionnaire locally, then they can download one from the Internet. For example, NGOs developed the CORE Group website for this. You can find a copy of an excellent questionnaire—KPC 2000+—at their website (http://www.coregroup.org/working_groups/monitoring.cfm) or (http://www.childsurvival.com/kpc2000/kpc2000.cfm).

C. Have the NGO change the questions it has found, if needed, to reflect the health messages of the project; these are the health messages written in Step A above. In addition, change the questions to reflect the correct gender and age group, if needed. The NGO's questionnaire should be as short as possible and designed to collect <u>only essential information</u> for planning and managing their program. This can be achieved if the NGO limits questions to those needed to measure its program indicators.

D. If the NGO cannot find a good question for measuring an indicator, this may mean the indicator is not measurable. If so, change the indicator and return to Step B above.

E. Once they prepare the questionnaire, the NGO may have to translate it into a local language. Translation has four steps.

(1) First, the questionnaire should be translated by a native speaker of the local language who also speaks and reads the language of the original questionnaire.

(2) Then other members of the team—health professionals who also speak and read the local language—must review the questionnaire. This is to decide whether the questions are clear.

(3) Then the questionnaire needs to be translated back into the original language of the first questionnaire. This is an important step to find out if the questions are correct and have kept the original meanings.

(4) Finally, the questionnaire has to be pre-tested. This means that you need to go to a local community, use the questionnaire and learn whether respondents understand the questions. If there are problems, the interviewee should work with the local respondent to form a clear question. Then this suggestion and others can be discussed and questions can be rewritten. **REMEMBER**, if you rewrite a question you have to pre-test it again.

TASK 5—Ask the NGO to identify all the participants that are taking part in the workshop.

Ask them to tell you which participants are associated with each SA. Sometimes an NGO assigns more than one person to an SA so the sampling and interviewing goes even quicker. Compare the number of participants with the number of SAs to be sure the NGO has identified enough people to take part in the training. Be sure the participants are committed to carrying out the sampling as soon as the training session is finished. And be sure that at least one participant assigned to an SA actually works there, or will work there—as the information s/he collects will be for him/her to use to manage the health program in the SA.

TASK 6—Prepare and send these materials to participants.

Send a description of logistical arrangements (for example, where the workshop is being held, where participants are staying), and the expected time of the workshop.

TASK 7—In the workshop, the trainer will need materials.

These days you can find sophisticated machines that make the training easier to carry out.

A. If you can use a computer and an LCD Powerpoint projector, arrange as soon as possible to have it available to you for the entire training and data-collection period. The overheads in this guide can be projected on a wall with an LCD Powerpoint machine. Be sure to have one or more electrical extension cord(s) and at least one extra light bulb available.

B. If an LCD Powerpoint machine is not available then get an overhead projector. Many schools or agencies have one. You can copy all the overheads included in the Participant's Manual onto transparencies (acetates). Be sure to have one or more electrical extension cord(s) and at least 1 extra light bulb available.

C. If neither overhead nor LCD Powerpoint projectors are available, the trainer must prepare flip-charts of each overhead. In addition, every training site—regardless of whether overheads or Powerpoint slides are available, should have flip-charts available. Have several of these, with several markers, since they have a tendency to dry up rapidly in a hot climate. They are also useful for the field exercises.

TASK 8—Copy all training materials, the participant's manual, and enough questionnaires for the field practice. Participants Manuals and Workbooks can be purchased from the publisher as cheaply as it is to photocopy them yourself.

Have all materials prepared and ready so you can focus on the training rather than solving a crisis because your materials are not ready for the participants to use.

Good luck with your community assessment!

MODULE ONE

Why should I do a survey and why should I use the LQAS method?

Session 1: **Introducing Participants and the Training/Survey**

Session 2: **Uses of Surveys**

Session 3: **Random Sampling**

Session 4: **Using LQAS Sampling for Surveys**

Session 5: **Using LQAS for Baseline Surveys**

MODULE ONE/Session 1: Introducing Participants and the Training/Survey

PURPOSE This is the opening session of the training. The purpose is to introduce the training and the survey—the overall schedule and the daily schedule—and yourself (training staff) and give participants the chance to introduce themselves and interact before getting into the actual content of the workshop (which begins in Session 2). You should also deal with any site logistics (meals, telephones, transportation, etc.) at this time.

TIME One hour to 90 minutes, depending on group size.

OBJECTIVES By the end of this session, participants will have:

1. Introduced themselves to each other.
2. Reviewed the overall schedule for the training and the survey, and also the daily schedule.
3. Asked any questions they have about logistics.

PREPARATION Before you begin this session, you will need to do the following:

1. Instruct the participating organization to organize the program site into about 5 supervision areas (see page x in the Introduction Section for a discussion on what supervision areas are). While more than 5 SAs is okay, although it requires more work than may be necessary, at least 3 or 4 are needed to use LQAS. Each supervisor would be in charge of about 2 dozen communities or health workers. These supervisors should be the participants of the workshop.
2. Request a list of all participant names and the name of their supervision area.

3. Direct the participating organization to prepare a list of all communities in each supervision area, with their estimated population size and detailed maps that will be included in the sampling (where available), or household lists (where available).
4. Prepare/adapt the participant interview overhead (Overhead #1) as necessary.
5. Prepare/adapt the purpose and skills statements (Overheads #2 and #3), the overview of the training (Overhead #4), and the daily schedule/agenda for the training and survey (Overhead #5) as necessary.
6. Prepare for the opening formalities (see STEP 1 below) as necessary.
7. Prepare the logistics presentation (see STEP 7 below).

DELIVERY

STEP 1—Conduct the opening formalities. This would normally include a few words of welcome by the training workshop leader and introducing any speakers/guests you may have invited to this session. These might include political or community leaders, donor officials, training sponsors, government officials, senior officials of your organization, or any other relevant people. These people will then make brief remarks.

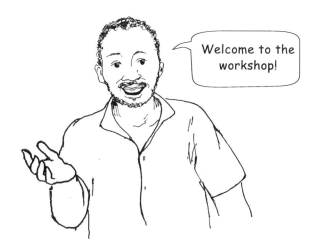

STEP 2—Introduce yourself. After speakers have left (or finished their remarks), introduce yourself.

STEP 3—Ask participants to interview each other. Display Overhead #1: Getting To Know One Another

(refer participants to their copy) which contains the questions participants should ask each other in their interview. If they wish, they can record answers on notebook paper. Explain that after the interviews you will ask each participant to introduce his or her partner.

STEP 4—Have participants introduce each other.

STEP 5—Review the overall design of the training.

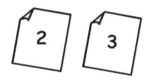

A. Display Overhead #2: Purpose of the LQAS Workshop and Overhead #3: Skills To Be Learned (refer participants to their copies) and go through each point.

B. Display Overhead #4: Overview of the LQAS Training (refer participants to their copy) and go over the 5 modules and 16 sessions listed there. You can also make a wall chart of this overhead and refer to it throughout the training. Participants like to see how far they have come and how far they have to go.

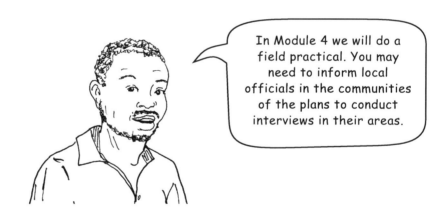

NOTE: For baseline surveys you will cover Modules 1-5, and for regular monitoring you will cover Modules 1-4 and 6. Explain the logic of the training, how it will unfold, and what participants will be doing as they complete each module.

STEP 6—Go over the training schedule/agenda. Display Overhead #5: Abbreviated Agenda for Modules 1-5 and 6.

Review both the daily schedule and the schedule for the entire training.

> **NOTE: A sample of a DETAILED VERSION OF THE AGENDA is in Appendix 1 of the guide. After adapting the sample to your needs, copies should be made for each trainer and participant and put into the "participant's manuals."**

STEP 7—Discuss training site and training logistics. If someone else gives this talk, it's a good idea for the lead trainer to review the presentation with the speaker ahead of time to make sure all the information is accurate and clearly organized. This can save many headaches later. We suggest that important details be provided to participants on a written handout.

> **SUGGESTION: You or someone else should explain all administrative and logistical arrangements, for the workshop and for the field visits (such as details of transportation, per diem, meals, lodging, equipment, supplies, etc.). It needs to be clear who the point person is for participants to discuss concerns and questions.**

STEP 8—Discussion of the field site where data will be collected.

A. Display Overhead #6: Defining Catchment Area and Supervision Areas. Managers will have already organized the catchment area for an NGO's program into supervision areas. Each supervision area will have several communities. Take a few minutes so a participant from the NGO can show the group on a map where their program catchment area is located, and where each of their supervision areas is located, too. Post a map on the wall of the training room with the catchment area and supervision area boundaries marked.

> **IMPORTANT: Use maps that are already available to show where the boundaries of the catchment area are; maps that show details about the terrain and roads are especially good to use. Now draw boundaries for each SA.**

If a map is not available, then draw one by hand. This is a good time to remind participants that they should have organized their program area into supervision areas by now!

B. On days 3 and 4 of the training, participants will go out to a field location to carry out practice exercises. Tell the participants where this will be and show them a map of the area. Also, make it clear who will be responsible for contacting the local leaders and making sure the map is accurate!

MODULE ONE/Session 2: Uses of Surveys

PURPOSE   The purpose of this session is to show participants what they will gain by going through this training. While they may understand in general the importance of having reliable information about the impact and results of their programs, many participants will not understand why they have to sit through a 4-day workshop on the subject of surveys. The point of this session, then, is to show them how they will be able to use the data that comes from surveys. It is expected that once trainees see how helpful survey data can be, they will recognize the value of and need for this training.

TIME   45–60 minutes.

OBJECTIVES   By the end of this session, participants will have:

1. Described why coverage is important to know.
2. Listed how surveys will help them in their work.
3. Analyzed coverage in different scenarios and made recommendations based on results.

DELIVERY   **STEP 1**—Define coverage. Display Overhead #7: What Is Coverage? and ask for responses. Be sure you or someone else defines coverage correctly.

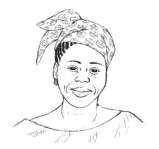

One of the key uses of surveys is to measure <u>coverage</u>. WHAT IS <u>COVERAGE</u>?

> **IMPORTANT: COVERAGE** is the percentage of people in any catchment area who either: (a) **know a recommended health behavior**; (b) **practice a recommended health behavior**; or who (c) **receive a particular service**.

STEP 2: Discuss why coverage is important.

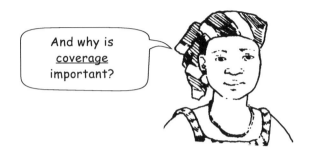

> **SUGGESTION: Be sure you or someone else makes the point that knowing the coverage—of various health knowledge and practices—helps us plan by allowing us to choose priorities. We can decide to focus our efforts on improving those health knowledge and practices that have low coverage. Over time, repeated measures of coverage show us if our efforts are leading to improvements in coverage. Additionally, knowing that the coverage is especially poor in one or more supervision areas helps us choose priorities. We can decide to focus our efforts in those supervision areas with poor coverage.**

To put it another way, knowing that coverage is poor in just a few supervision areas shows where you have pockets of risk and where you have to focus your efforts to reduce health risks.

STEP 3—Explain the results of measuring coverage. Display Overhead #8: What Surveys Can Show You and discuss the two points.

> **POINT ONE: Make sure you or someone else explains that when a survey reveals LARGE differences in coverage among supervision areas, this identifies the areas that are not doing well and, all other things being equal, should be your priority.**

This usually means that you should focus your attention, resources and especially your time, on your priority areas.

> **POINT TWO:** Then explain that when the data from a survey reveal LITTLE difference in coverage among supervision areas, this tells you that you are having the same succes (or lack of) in all areas. This would normally mean that you could continue to treat all areas the same.

(Naturally, if the survey shows that coverage is uniformly poor, then this means that the program may need to be redesigned to improve its impact. This may also mean that all areas need more resources. If it shows that coverage is uniformly good, then other interventions can be selected as priorities even as the current one is maintained.)

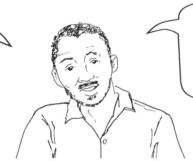

And in conclusion . . . without knowing coverage—and if it is different in the various supervision areas—we will not know how to make the best use of our resources!

. . . and without doing surveys, you can't know coverage. And all of this is especially crucial when resources are <u>limited</u>!

STEP 4—Conduct the "three scenarios" exercise. Explain that participants will now do an exercise that illustrates the points just made about surveys and coverage. Continue in the following manner:

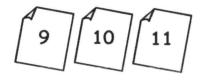

A. Divide participants into <u>groups of 3-4 people</u> and explain that each group will work on a different scenario.

B. Display Overheads #9, #10, and #11, the NGO Program Area scenarios (refer participants to their copies). Assign one scenario to each group. Be sure that each of the three scenarios has been assigned to a group.

Module 1, Session 2

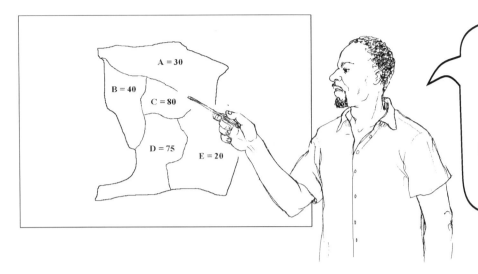

C. Display Overhead #12: Using Survey Data (refer participants to their copy).

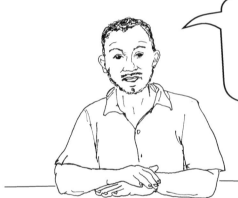

D. Give participants <u>20 minutes</u> to discuss the data from their scenarios and answer the four questions.

> **See answer guide for correct answers to OVERHEAD #12**

E. Ask for a brief summary of their answer to question 4: What might you propose to do about HIV/AIDS in the program area? Ask a volunteer from each scenario to describe their group's conversation. Ask why the group decided to propose these particular actions.

F. If the group "got the point," that surveys help us set priorities, move on to the next session in this module. If they did not, try to find out where the group went wrong and correct any misunderstanding. (Better yet, ask other participants to correct the misunderstanding.) Display Overhead #13: Uses of Surveys to summarize the main points of this session.

Answer Guide for Overhead 12
(Note: This answer guide should not appear in the participant's guide)

Using Survey Data

Indicator: Percent of women (15-49) who know at least two ways to prevent HIV transmission

	Possible Scenarios		
Supervision Area	Scenario One (1) True Coverage (%)	Scenario Two (2) True Coverage (%)	Scenario Three (3) True Coverage (%)
A	30	85	25
B	40	80	20
C	80	90	30
D	75	85	25
E	20	80	20

Analysis:

Look only at the true coverage figures within your assigned scenario (1, 2 or 3):

1. Discuss for a few minutes the differences in coverage among the 5 supervision areas *within your scenario*:
   - What is the difference in coverage among the 5 supervision areas?
   scenario 1=60%; scenario 2=10%; scenario 3=10%
   - How great is the difference? Very different? Little difference?
   1=very different; 2=little difference; 3=little difference

2. Does coverage for the overall program area appear MIXED, HIGH, LOW?   **1=MIXED; 2=HIGH; 3=LOW**

3. What may be possible reasons for why, in your scenario, the program area has this coverage? **Discussion**

4. What might you propose to do about HIV/AIDS in the program area? **Discussion**

12   Module 1, Session 2

MODULE ONE/Session 3: Random Sampling

PURPOSE The purpose of this session is to explain random sampling as a survey technique and to show how it is carried out and why it works.

To introduce this session, you will need to explain to participants that there is more than one way to collect the information they used in their scenario in the previous session (Session 2). You can interview *all* the women in the program area and ask them if they know ways to prevent HIV transmission. Or you can take what is called a random *sample*, interviewing fewer people and using their answers to give you a good idea of what women know. Obviously, interviewing every woman in the catchment area would be time-consuming and costly and is not practical in many situations. Random sampling, however, makes it possible to get useful data more quickly and with less effort and cost.

TIME 45 minutes.

OBJECTIVES By the end of this session, participants will have:

1. Contrasted using a census versus a sampling approach to gaining information.
2. Described problems with non-random sampling.
3. Committed to using random sampling during their fieldwork.

PREPARATION 1. You will need to prepare two bags of marbles or painted stones of the same size—drafts (checkers) or poker chips also work well. The first bag of marbles should have 50 green and 50 red marbles (or any two other colors). The second bag should have 80 green and 20 red marbles. You may want to have a towel for the demonstration. Place the marbles on it so they don't roll away.

2. You should also prepare the sign-up sheet described in STEP 6 below. At the top of this sign-up sheet, write the following: "I commit to using random sampling throughout this survey and will ask questions whenever I need help."

DELIVERY   **STEP 1**—Demonstrate random sampling. Using the bags of marbles, lead participants through a demonstration of how to take a sample.

> **IMPORTANT: Complete these exercises one step at a time.**

A. Sit in the center of the group (at a table or on the ground) with participants in a circle around you.

B. Show participants both bags of marbles.

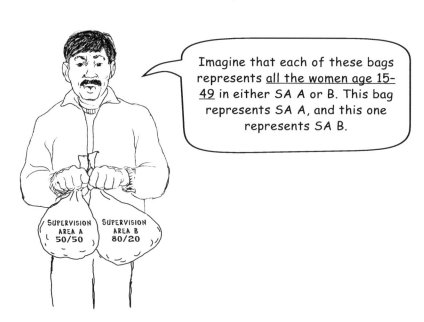

C. Explain that a green marble represents a woman (15–49) in an area who knows at least two ways to prevent HIV transmission and a red marble represents a woman (15–49) in the same supervision area (15–49) who does not know at least two ways to prevent HIV transmission.

> **GREEN = women who know**
> **RED = women who DO NOT know**

D. Explain how we learn how many or what percentage of women know at least two ways to prevent HIV transmission.

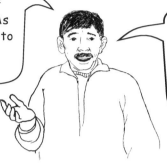

Now, we want to know what percentage of women in these 2 SAs know 2 or more ways to prevent HIV transmission.

One way to get the answer would be to count ALL the green and red marbles in the bags, but let's assume we do not have the time or money to do this. Instead, we could select a SAMPLE of the women from each supervision area.

E. Ask for a volunteer to take a sample of 30 marbles from bag A (the 50/50 bag representing supervision area A) and put them into a small bowl or container.

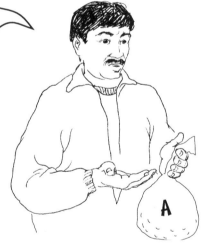
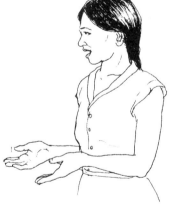

Could I please have a volunteer? FIRST, with your eyes closed, please take 30 marbles from the bag. NEXT, count, in a loud voice, the number of marbles you remove as you put them into the container.

F. Then ask the volunteer to count the marbles and write these numbers on a flip-chart or where they can be seen by all. Remind participants that green marbles stand for women who know at least two ways to prevent HIV transmission and red marbles stand for women who do not.

Module 1, Session 3   15

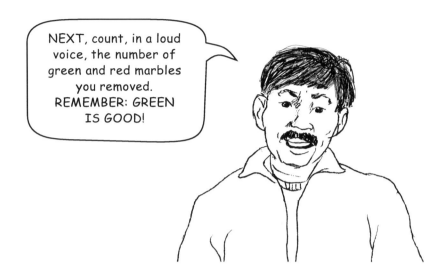

G. Now ask the group to answer this question:

> **QUESTION: "Using this sample, would you say that most women in supervision area A (show the bag) know at least two ways to prevent HIV transmission; that few women do; or that somewhere in between 'most' and 'few' women do?"**
> **ANSWER should be "somewhere in between."**

H. Now ask the volunteer to count the marbles remaining in the bag and state the total number of green and red marbles.

I. Ask the group how the sample of marbles compares to the count of all marbles.

> **SUGGESTION: After the volunteer counts the marbles remaining in the bag, ask the group if they think the sample correctly describes the contents of the bag.**

STEP 2—Repeat the demonstration with bag B (representing supervision area B). You can omit this step if the group has caught on (but you should probably not skip it if the first demonstration did not "work.")

STEP 3—Demonstrate *non*-random sampling. Participants should understand why the sampling they do as part of LQAS must be random—and why non-random sampling does not yield reliable information on which to base program decisions. This demonstration will make the point effectively.

   A. Empty the 50/50 bag of marbles on the ground/floor/table where all participants can see them.

> **SUGGESTION: It is helpful to place the marbles onto a rough surface (such as a towel) to prevent them from rolling away.**

   B. Create a pretend community using marbles to represent women living in a different house. Separate the green marbles from the red, and place the green marbles near you and the red marbles just out of your reach.

   C. Explain that you will pretend to be a program official who has been asked to do a survey. The purpose of the survey is to find out what percentage of women in a given supervision area know at least two ways to prevent HIV transmission.

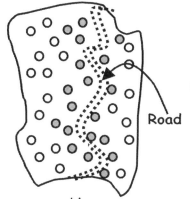

● = green marbles
O = red marbles

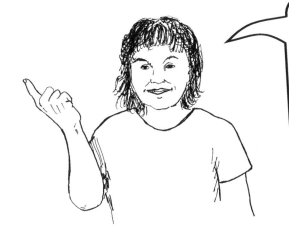

In this community, some of the women are EASIER to interview because they live NEXT TO THE ROAD (point to the green marbles near you and, if possible, arrange them in a line that borders an imaginary road) while other women live in remote areas and are harder to reach and interview (indicate the red pile, scattering them at further distances from you).

   D. Explain that it has just started to rain in the village and you have decided all the women in the supervision area are alike. Therefore, you do

Module 1, Session 3

not need to interview any women in the remote areas. You will just interview women who live close to a road, and save much time and money and stay out of the rain. And the information will be "just as good."

E. Take a few green marbles from the line near the imaginary road, counting them aloud. Then announce that the survey findings show that all or most women in the supervision area know at least two ways to prevent HIV transmission.

F. Explain the "results" of the sample, still acting as the pretend program official.

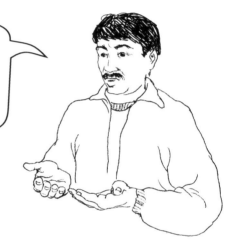

Finally, from my sample, I can tell that HIV/AIDS should <u>not</u> be a problem in this supervision area, so we can spend our money on other interventions.

Ask participants if they agree. <u>They should disagree, but ask them to explain why.</u>

STEP 4—Debrief the demonstration you have just completed. Ask participants their reaction to the demonstration.

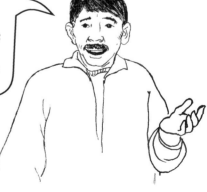

How are the results different from the random sample taken from the same bag? Why are they different? Are conclusions and program decisions based on this non-random sample going to be reliable?

STEP 5—Reiterate the advantages of sampling. Display Overhead #14: Why Random Sample? (refer participants to their handout) and review the contents. Be sure to repeat the main advantage. (Alternative: Ask participants to state the advantages of random sampling *before* you post the overhead.)

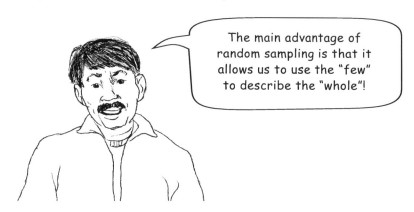

STEP 6—Invite participants to commit to random sampling. Post a sheet of flip-chart paper on the wall (prepared earlier), numbered from "1" through the total number of participants. Assure participants that this list of names is to be displayed during this training, and it will not be shown to anyone else or used outside this training room.

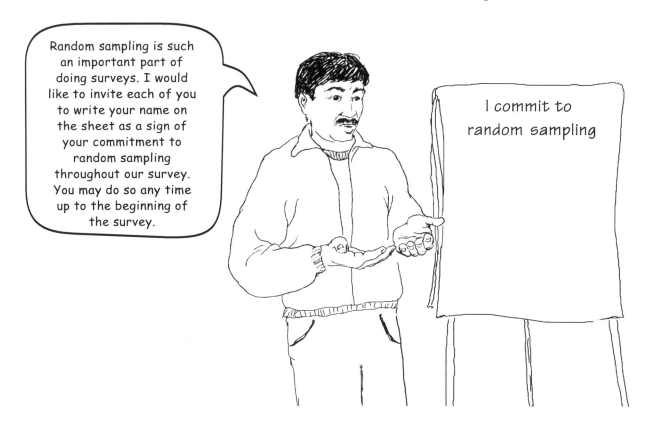

Module 1, Session 3

MODULE ONE/Session 4: Using LQAS Sampling for Surveys

PURPOSE This session introduces the LQAS technique. To introduce the session, relate it to the random sampling session just completed. Explain that now we are going to introduce a special type of random sampling called LQAS. It is an approach that allows us to use small random samples to distinguish between supervision areas with high and low coverage. Using small samples makes conducting surveys more efficient for busy program people.

TIME One hour.

OBJECTIVES By the end of this session, participants will have:

1. Practiced LQAS sampling on their own.
2. Described how a sample size of 19 is satisfactory to distinguish between high and low coverage in a supervision area.

PREPARATION Before beginning this session, do the following:

1. Prepare a bag of 100 marbles—50 green + 50 red—for every three participants in the class.
2. Prepare a second bag of 100 marbles—80 green + 20 red—for every three participants.
   (You may use an alternative to marbles, such as painted stones, drafts/checkers or poker chips. However, the alternative item must come in two distinct colors and each piece must be the same size and shape as other pieces. This is so each piece is indistinguishable by touch from the other pieces.)
3. For each group of three participants, bring a bag or jar or some other receptacle to hold marbles.

DELIVERY **STEP 1**—Put this session in context. If necessary, briefly display Overhead #4 from Module One/Session 1 Overview of the LQAS Training. Do this to remind participants where they are and where this session fits into the overall design of this training.

STEP 2—Introduce the topic. Using language like that in PURPOSE above, explain that we are now going to show LQAS sampling.

IMPORTANT PRINCIPLE: Remind participants that the overall goal we are all aiming for is to <u>make the best use of limited resources by setting priorities</u>, for indicators and for supervision areas, and that the LQAS technique presented in this session is one of the most efficient ways to collect the coverage information needed to establish such priorities.

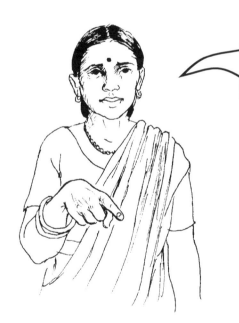

For the purpose of setting priorities, we need only to distinguish areas that reach "coverage targets" from those that do not. "Coverage targets," means the level of coverage—a specific percent of the population—you had earlier decided to reach by the time of the survey. The ability to distinguish areas that reach coverage targets from those that do not is precisely the reason LQAS was developed. If we find this situation, we can give special attention to areas that have not yet met our coverage targets.

A defining characteristic of LQAS is that it uses a sample size of 19 for each SA. In this session we will demonstrate that 19 is sufficient to distinguish between high and low coverage.

STEP 3—Demonstrate LQAS sampling. Complete a demonstration of the LQAS technique as follows:

A. Display Overhead #15: NGO Program Area – Scenario 4 (refer participants to their handout).

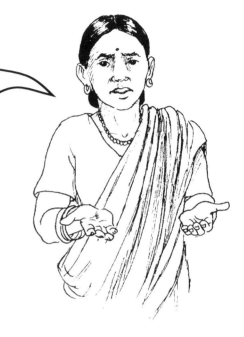

Again, we are working with a fictitious NGO Program Area, the same that was used in Session 2. As you can see, we do not know the coverage for TWO of the FIVE supervision Areas, SA A and SA C, for the indicator "percentage of women (15-49) who know at least two ways to prevent HIV transmission." Because we want to make decisions about deploying our program resources, we will need to do a survey of these two areas to see whether or not they need special attention.

B. Explain how we will do the survey.

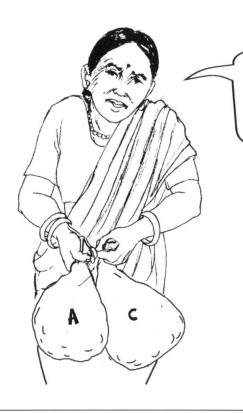

We don't know the coverage in SA "A" or "C" so we will do a survey interviewing 19 women from each of the 2 SAs. We will demonstrate that this is adequate for our purposes of identifying priority areas.

C. Show participants the bag of marbles for Supervision Area A (with 50 green and 50 red marbles). Explain that the marbles in this bag represent all the women (15–49) in this area. The green marbles represent all the women who know at least two ways to prevent HIV transmission. The red marbles represent those women who do not.

> **HINT: You can place the bag of marbles on top of area A on the overhead to emphasize this point.**

D. Explain how they will sample these bags. Display Overhead #16: LQAS Sampling Results.

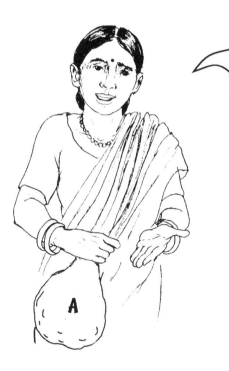

> First we are going to take 5 samples of 19 from SA A (show bag), and then you will do the same with SA C (show bag). You will record the results on OVERHEAD 16: LQAS Sampling Results, and I will record the group results here.

E. Take the first sample from the bag for Area A, removing 19 marbles a few at a time, and place them in a clear jar (or some other receptacle).

> **HINT: Begin by shaking the marbles in the bag to ensure that they are randomly mixed. You can comment again on the importance of random sampling.**

Module 1, Session 4

F. Count the green marbles in the jar (women who know at least two ways to prevent HIV transmission). Write the number on Overhead #16 under the # Correct column, Area A, on the line for Sample 1. Ask participants to record this number in the same place on their copy of the overhead. <u>Then return the 19 marbles to their original bag.</u>

G. Divide participants into small groups. Give each group an Area A type bag (with 50 green and 50 red marbles) and a receptacle. Ask each group to repeat this same process: 1) Take the first, second, third, fourth and fifth samples from the Area A bag. 2) Count the number of green marbles in each sample. 3) Record the # correct on their own copy of the overhead.

> **SUGGESTION: Once the groups have finished, the trainer should write the # correct from the subsequent samples of the groups on an overhead, so that all five lines on the overhead are filled in. Then wait a moment before discussing the results.**

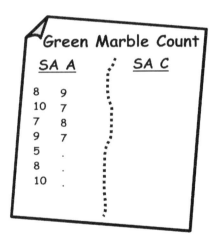

H. After each group has finished taking five samples of 19 marbles and recorded the number of green marbles, ask each group to report their results to the large group. The trainer will record all these results on a single overhead or flip-chart page (see figure to left). Save this sheet to continue the demonstration in STEP 3-J.

I. Now ask each group to count the total number of green marbles in the entire bag. Enter this number as the numerator in the "verify" space for SA-A on Overhead #16. Also ask them to count the <u>total number of green and red</u> marbles in the bag. Enter this number as the denominator in the "verify" space for SA-A and then calculate the percentage of marbles that are green.

> **IMPORTANT: Verify that each group concludes that 50% of the marbles are green.**

J. Give each group a bag for Area C (80 green and 20 red marbles). (Once again, the trainer should record # correct on an overhead or flipchart page from each of the five samples from each group. Save this sheet to continue the demonstration in STEP 6.)

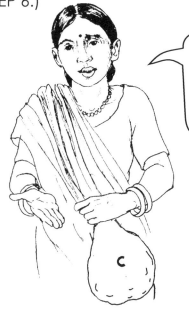

Now, do the same thing for SA C. Repeat the entire process—take five samples and complete the lines on Overhead #16 for SA C.

K. Repeat the process described in E above. This time, however, each group should decide that 80% of the marbles are green.

STEP 4—Show how to find the decision rule for the Area A samples in the following manner:

A. Display Overhead #17: The LQAS Table and explain what the columns and rows mean.

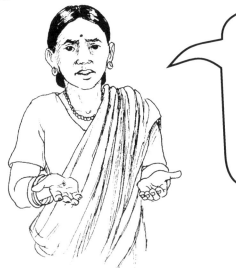

Let me explain how this table works. The first column (far left) is the size of your sample. Samples 12–30 are displayed. The percentages across the top of the page represent coverage targets (which are used for program monitoring and evaluation, but not relevant for baseline surveys) or average coverage (which is used for baseline, monitoring and evaluation surveys). Baselines will be explained later.

Module 1, Session 4

B. Show how to find the decision rule. The decision rule is the minimum number of people who must have received an intervention to conclude safely that a supervision area has reached average or target coverage.

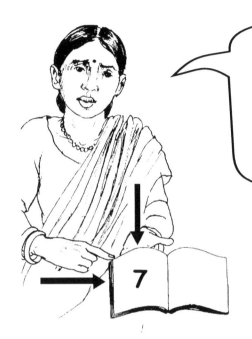

Now we will use this table to find a <u>decision rule</u>. Select the percentage column that is your target (we are using 50% for Area A) and go down that column until you come to the row with your sample size (in this case 19); the number that appears at the spot where the column and the row cross (<u>7 in this example</u>) is the decision rule (or minimum number for decision-making purposes).

C. Use the sheet with the sampling results for all the groups for both SA A and C. Ask the participants to inspect the # correct for each of the samples from <u>Area A</u> and whether it is seven or more. Circle the cases that are <u>fewer than 7</u> (if there are any) (see figure below). In almost all the samples, the number correct will be at least seven green marbles.

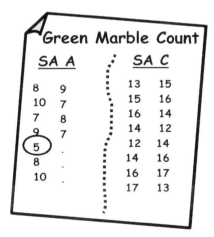

STEP 5—Find the decision rule for the samples from SA C. Repeat the process described under STEP 4 above with SA C samples. Since 80% of the marbles are green, the coverage is 80%. Using overhead #17, the groups should find that the decision rule is 13 green marbles. Reviewing the group's sampling of the SA C bag, participants should find that for almost all samples, at least 13 marbles were green in each of their samples of 19. This is because the decision rule is 13. The trainer should circle all cases (if there are any) where the sample was <u>fewer than 13</u> in the SA C bag.

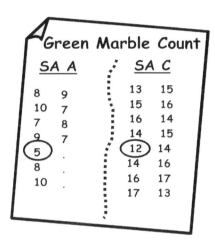

STEP 6—Using the sheet, ask participants to compare the results of Areas A and C.

    A. Tell participants that the LQAS table decision rules will lead participants to make the correct decision at least 90% of the time. In other words, for SAs that have 50% coverage, such as Area A, you have 7 or more green marbles more than 90% of the time. Ask participants how many times in the exercise there were fewer than 7 green marbles. This almost never happened. Therefore, the LQAS table almost always identified Supervision Areas with 50% coverage.

    B. Now ask them how many times Area C, with 80% coverage, had fewer than 13 green marbles. Show them that this never or almost never happened. Therefore, the LQAS Table almost always identified Supervision Areas with 80% coverage.

Module 1, Session 4

C. Now ask participants how many times in Area A there were 13 or more green marbles. This almost never happened either. Almost all 50% bag samples should have fewer than 13. And, almost all 80% bag samples should have at least 13. Therefore, areas with 50% coverage almost never would be confused with areas with high coverage, such as 80%.

IMPORTANT POINT: Point out that Area A would never or almost never be mistakenly classified as an area with high coverage like Area C.

D. Make the point (or have a participant do so):

IMPORTANT POINT: Once average coverage has been measured or a target coverage has been selected, you can easily determine whether the average coverage or target has or hasn't been reached with a sample size of 19.

STEP 7—End with a review. Display Overhead #18: What a Sample of 19 Can Tell Us, Overhead #19: What a Sample of 19 Cannot Tell Us, and Overhead #20: Why Use a Random Sample of 19? Go over the points with participants.

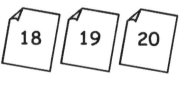

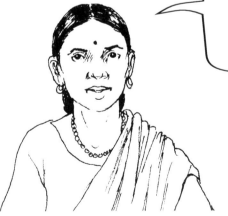

In conclusion, let's review:
- what a sample of 19 can tell us,
- what a sample of 19 can NOT tell us,
- why we use a sample of 19.

MODULE ONE/Session 5: Using LQAS for Baseline Surveys

PURPOSE The LQAS method can be used for various purposes. The previous session showed the basic soundness of the LQAS approach (that 19 is a large enough sample size for most surveys). In this exercise we show how to use the LQAS technique to decide 3 things: (1) Whether a supervision area has above or below average coverage for a particular indicator (STEPs 1 and 2); (2) Which indicators *within* a supervision area are doing well and which are not (STEP 3); and (3) How supervision areas within a program area compare with one another (STEP 4)—3 of the principal uses of a baseline and monitoring survey.

TIME 45 minutes.

OBJECTIVES By the end of this session, participants will have:

1. Compared how using LQAS for baseline surveys is different from using LQAS for program monitoring.
2. Calculated coverage.
3. Compared indicators across supervision areas.
4. Used coverage data to help them make program decisions.

DELIVERY **STEP 1**—Demonstrate use of LQAS at baseline to assess whether or not a supervision area is below-average coverage for a particular indicator.

A. Display Overhead #21: Five Supervision Areas and One Indicator.

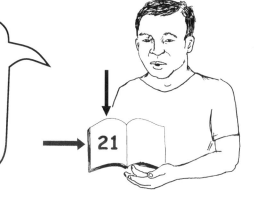

This overhead contains data for this indicator for all five SAs (collected through LQAS sampling). Let's determine if an SA has above- or below-average coverage for the indicator "women who know at least 2 ways to prevent HIV transmission."

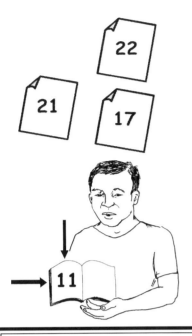

B. Display Overhead #22: LQAS Concepts for Baseline Surveys and review the meaning of Average Coverage and Decision Rule.

C. Explain how average coverage is calculated (refer to question 1 on Overhead #21, below the chart), resulting in this case with a figure of 65.3%. Explain that this is the reason 65.3% is written in the space provided in Overhead #21 for the Coverage Estimate.

D. Answer question 2 on Overhead #21, "What is the Decision Rule?" by showing how the LQAS summary table (Module One/Session 4/ Overhead #17) was used to arrive at the number "11."

IMPORTANT PRINCIPLE: Display the LQAS chart again, put your finger on the top row and find 70%. (Explain that for purposes of using this chart, we always round up the coverage figure, 65.3% in this case, to the next highest 5% increment, 70% in this example.) Now move your finger down the 70% column until it meets the horizontal row for the sample size of 19. Where the column and the row cross, your finger will be on number 11. This means that as long as there were <u>11 or more</u> correct answers to the indicator, coverage is not below average.

E. Show how question 3, "Is coverage below average?" was answered for each SA by noting whether the # correct was 11 or above, or below 11, for each SA.

> **See answer guide for correct answers to OVERHEAD #21**

F. Ask participants to answer questions 4 and 5.

> **See answer guide for correct answers to OVERHEAD #21**

30   Module 1, Session 5

STEP 2—Have participants do the second example (display Overhead #23: Five Supervision Areas and One Indicator: Participant Worksheet) on their own copy of the practice sheet.

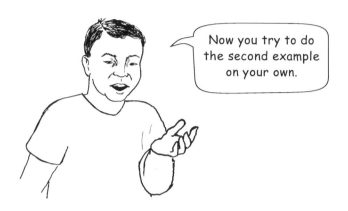

Then go over the example with them to see if they have done it correctly or have any questions.

> See answer guide for correct answers to OVERHEAD #23

STEP 3—Demonstrate using LQAS to assess the values of various indicators within the same supervision area.

> **IMPORTANT POINT:** After information has been gathered for a number of indicators, it is possible to use LQAS to determine which indicators within a particular supervision area are reaching average coverage and which are not, thus making it possible for a supervisor to know which indicators to focus on in his/her area

A. Display Overhead #24: Supervision Area A and Five Indicators (refer participants to their copy) and work through it with participants. Point out that this chart deals with Supervision Area A only.

B. Explain that for indicator 1 of Area A the average coverage was calculated in STEP 2 of this session. The number 6 was likewise determined to be the decision rule (having rounded the average upward to 45%). They can then see that the number correct is 7, which exceeds the decision rule. Therefore, they judge that Area A is at least of average coverage, and put "Y" in the last column.

C. Now have participants work through the other four indicators, filling in the boxes. They will need to keep the LQAS Summary Table handy (Module One/ Session 4/Overhead #17).

D. Go over the two questions below the chart.

> **See answer guide for correct answers to OVERHEAD #24**

STEP 4—Demonstrate using LQAS results to compare the baseline conditions of all supervision areas within one program area.

A. Display Overhead #25 Comparing Supervision Areas A, B, C, D & E (refer participants to their copy).

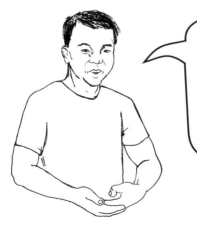

> By bringing together results from previous STEPs, we can now take a look at our entire program area and see which supervision areas are doing well overall and which need support. This chart combines the information gathered in STEPs 2 & 3.

B. Begin by filling in the three empty boxes for indicator 1. Participants will have to go back to their handout of Overhead #23 from STEP 2 above. Note what has been recorded in the far-right column for Areas A, B, and C, and transfer this information to this handout.

C. Now that the chart is complete, have participants answer the four questions at the bottom.

> **See the answer guide for correct answers to OVERHEAD #25**

STEP 5—End this Session.

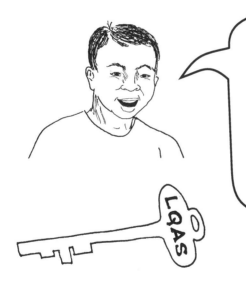

This session has shown how to use LQAS for baseline surveys. However, using LQAS for regular monitoring is the most common use of LQAS. The procedures for analyzing the data collected in supervision areas is slightly different. Using LQAS for monitoring programs is explained in a later session (Module 6.) Nevertheless, you know enough about LQAS now to collect LQAS data and understand what it tells you.

Answer Guide for Overhead 21
(Note: This answer guide should not appear in the participant's manual)

Five Supervision Areas & One Indicator

SUPERVISION AREA: A, B, C, D or E			
Indicator: Women who know 2 or more ways to prevent HIV transmission	# Correct	Average Coverage Estimate = **65.3%** Decision Rule = **11**	Equal to or Above Average? Yes or No
Supervision Area A	12		Yes
Supervision Area B	9		No
Supervision Area C	16		Yes
Supervision Area D	11		Yes
Supervision Area E	14		Yes

1. Add Number Correct in all SAs: 12 + 9 + 16 + 11 + 14 = **62**
   Add all Samples Sizes: 19 + 19 + 19 + 19 + 19 = **95**
   Coverage Estimate = Average Coverage = 62/95 = **65.3%** = **70%**
   (Round upward to the nearest interval of 5 to find the Decision Rule)

2. Use table to find Decision Rule. **Decision Rule = 11**

3. Is coverage in SAs generally equal to or above average? Yes or No?
   YES

4. Can you identify Supervision Areas that are your priorities? **YES**

   If yes which are they? If not, why can't you identify them? **Supervision Area B**

Answer Guide for Overhead 23
(Note: This answer guide should not appear in the participant's manual)

Five Supervision Areas & One Indicator: Participant Worksheet – For Baseline Surveys

Indicator: Women who used condoms each time with intercourse	# Correct	Average Coverage Estimate =	Equal to or Above Average? Yes or No
Supervision Area A	7	**45%**	Yes
Supervision Area B	3		No
Supervision Area C	2	Decision Rule (Using the LQAS Table) =	No
Supervision Area D	13		Yes
Supervision Area E	14	**6**	Yes

Questions:

1. For baseline surveys, add number correct in all SAs:

    7 + 3 + 2 + 13 + 14 = 39

    Add all sample sizes: <u>19</u> + <u>19</u> + <u>19</u> + <u>19</u> + <u>19</u> = **95**

    Average coverage = <u>   39   </u> / <u>   95   </u> = <u> **41.05% = 45%** </u>

2. What is the Decision Rule? **Decision Rule = 6**

3. Is coverage in SAs generally equal to or above average? Yes or No? **YES, or Somewhere in the Middle**

4. Can you identify Supervision Areas that are your priorities? **YES**

5. If yes, which are they? If not, why can't you identify them? **SA B and C**

Module 1, Session 5

Answer Guide for Overhead 24
(Note: This answer guide should not appear in the participant's manual)

Supervision Area A & Five Indicators

	Indicators	# Correct	Coverage Estimate	Decision Rule	Equal to or Above? Yes or No
1	Women who used condoms each time with intercourse	7	45%	6	YES
2	Men who used condoms each time with intercourse	4	20%	1	YES
3	Women who know how HIV is transmitted	4	45%	6	NO
4	Men who know how HIV is transmitted	13	65%	10	YES
5	Women who know where to get tested for HIV	6	30%	3	YES

Questions:

1. Can you identify indicators that are your priorities? **YES**

2. If yes, which indicators are they? If not, why can't you identify them?
   Indicator 3

Answer Guide for Overhead 25
(Note: This answer guide should not appear in the participant's manual)

Comparing Supervision Areas A, B, C, D, & E For Baseline Survey

	Indicators	Supervision Area				
		A	B	C	D	E
1	Women who used condoms each time with intercourse	Y	N	N	Y	Y
2	Men who used condoms each time with intercourse	Y	Y	Y	N	Y
3	Women who know how HIV is transmitted	N	N	Y	N	Y
4	Men who know how HIV is transmitted	Y	Y	N	N	Y
5	Women who know where to get tested for HIV	Y	Y	Y	N	Y

Questions:

1. Which Supervision Area(s) appears to be performing the best for all 5 indicators: A, B, C, D, or E? **E and maybe A**

2. Which SA(s) appears to need the most support for their overall program: A, B, C, D, or E? **D and maybe B and C**

3. Which indicator(s) needs improvement across most of the catchment area? **3 SAs are weak for Indicator 3.**

4. Which indicator(s) needs improvement in only a few SAs? **Indicator 1 and 4 (2 weak SAs); Indicator 2 and 5 (1 weak SA)**

5. For these weaker indicators:
   - Which SA(s) needs special attention? **D and maybe B and C**
   - Which SA(s) would you visit to learn possible ways to improve these weaker indicators? **E and possibly A**

MODULE TWO

Where should I conduct my survey?

Session 1: Identifying Interview Locations

MODULE TWO/Session 1: Identifying Interview Locations

PURPOSE Now that participants are committed to random sampling and persuaded of the validity and usefulness of LQAS, they are ready to apply the LQAS approach in a survey. The first step in a survey is to identify the locations of the 19 sets of interviews that will eventually be carried out. Identifying these locations is the subject of this session.

TIME 90 minutes.

OBJECTIVES By the end of this session, participants will have:

1. Calculated the cumulative population of a list of communities.
2. Calculated a sampling interval for 19 interviews.
3. Used a random number chart to define a random starting place for selecting communities.
4. Identified the location for 19 interviews using a random approach.

PREPARATION NOTE 1: For a Training of Trainers (TOT), move to DELIVERY STEP 1.
NOTE 2: For the participants' training, prepare the following:

1. Copies of the sampling frames developed with the managers during the TOT.
2. Adapt the following steps to cover the process used to develop the sampling frame with the managers. STEP 6 is important for participants to cover.

DELIVERY

STEP 1—Display Overhead #4 of Module One/Session 1 again (Overview of the LQAS Training Program) and show participants where we are in the overall design of the training.

STEP 2—Introduce the topic of this session: identifying interview locations. Display Overhead #1: Identifying Locations for Interviews (refer participants to their copy) and explain the next step.

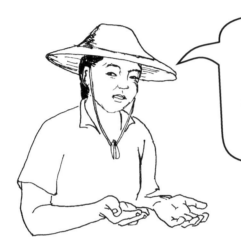

Now we are going to put LQAS to use in a sample survey that we will begin working on in this session. These are the five steps (refer to Overhead 1). We will now go through this process in order to identify actual interview locations.

HINT: (If population figures are not available for this session, then find any other information that reflects the different size of communities or neighborhoods. The total number of houses is often a good substitute for population size.)

If no information is available then try to learn what the relative sizes of the communities are. See if you can determine if one community is one-and-a-half times greater than another, or 2 times greater, etc.

STEP 3—Show the first step on the overhead: list communities and their total population. Display Overhead #2: List of Communities and Total Population for a fictitious supervision area (refer participants to their copy of this list).

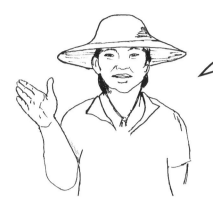

This is a list of communities in an SA, each shown with an estimated population. In the case of an urban area, we may have data for neighborhoods. For survey purposes we need to know only the total population of each community/neighborhood, not how many men vs. women, for example, or adults vs. children.

STEP 4—Show the second step: calculate the cumulative population.

A. Display Overhead #3: Calculate the Cumulative Population (refer participants to their copy).

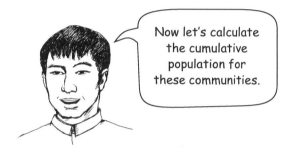

Now let's calculate the cumulative population for these communities.

Begin by adding the population of the second community (Santai, **730**) to that of the first (Pagai, **548**) and writing the total (**548 + 730 = 1278**) in the first blank space in the far-right column, "Cumulative Population."

B. Repeat this process by adding the population of the third community (Serina, **686**) to that of the combined population of Pagai and Santai (**1278**) to get the new total (**686 + 1278 = 1964**). Write it in the blank space in the far-right column. Then do the same for the next community, Mulrose, adding its population (**280**) to the previous total (**1964**) to get the new total: **280 + 1964 = 2244**.

C. Now let participants practice by filling in the 10 remaining blank lines at the bottom of the chart. When everyone is finished, have them call out their answers as you fill in the ten blank lines on your overhead.

STEP 5—Explain the third step in Overhead #1: calculate the sampling interval.

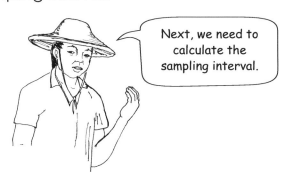

Next, we need to calculate the sampling interval.

Display Overhead #4: Calculate the Sampling Interval, and take participants through this step, filling in the blank at the bottom of the overhead. The answer is **23489/19 = 1236.26**.

STEP 6—Show the fourth step: choose a random number. Explain that choosing random numbers is a common task when conducting a survey using a random approach.

> **REMIND the group why RANDOM is important, and refer to the commitment sheet which they have had the chance to sign.**

In this particular instance we are using a random number to help us identify interview locations. Display Overhead #5: A Random Number Table (refer participants to their copy) that has 14 columns made up of rows of random numbers. You can use any randomizing process you wish, but using a random-number table is recommended.

    A. Restate the number of the sampling interval (1236.26) fixed in the previous step.

    B. Explain that the random number has to be between 1 and the sampling interval, 1236. (The decimal point is not used in this step.)

    C. Identify the highest possible number of digits in the random number, which in this case is 4, the number of digits in the interval (1...2...3...6).

D. Displaying Overhead #5: Random Number Table, you will now explain how to use it. First, notice that each row of random numbers has five digits. Have participants decide which of the five displayed on the table they will use in this particular case. (You should recommend that they use the first four digits. Then draw a line through the fifth column to eliminate it. That is why in the figure below you see only four digits.)

E. Now ask participants to close their eyes and hold a pencil in the air over the random-number table. Then ask them to bring the pencil down on the table while keeping their eyes closed. The pencil should strike on or near a row of random numbers near one of the columns of numbers. Using the first four digits, ask participants whether the number is in the range of 1 to 1236. If it is not, have them move to the next row, and ask them to keep doing this until they find a 4-digit number in this range. When they do, that number is a random number that could be used in this example. <u>Let's assume the random number selected is **0622**</u>.

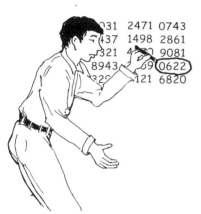

STEP 7—Explain the fifth and final step in this process: using a random number and sampling interval to identify locations of 19 interviews. Participants are now ready to combine the results of the third and fourth steps of this process to identify interview locations. Display Overhead #6: Identify the Location of Each of the 19 Interviews in a Supervision Area: Worksheet.

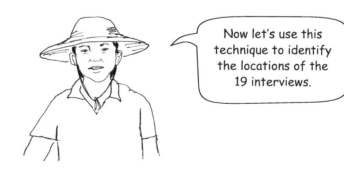

Now let's use this technique to identify the locations of the 19 interviews.

SUGGESTION: Take participants through the process for the first four interview locations.

Module 2, Session 1   43

A. Pointing to Overhead #6 row 1, explain:
The location number of the **first interview is the random number**. For this demonstration, we are assuming that **random number 622** was selected in the previous step.

> **IMPORTANT POINT:** The location of the <u>first interview</u> is the first community on the list with a cumulative population equal to or larger than the random number. In other words, find the community on Overhead #7 in which the 622nd person is located, Santai.

B. Pointing to Overhead #6 row 2, explain that the location number of the <u>second interview</u> is equal to the random number plus the sampling interval, in this case 622 + 1236.26 = 1858.26 (for this step you always use the decimal).

> **HINT:** Now go to <u>Overhead #7</u>. The location of the <u>second interview</u> will be the first community on the list with a cumulative population equal to or larger than 1858 (note: the decimal is NOT used for identifying the location).

C. Pointing to Overhead #6 row 3, explain that the location number of the <u>third interview</u> is equal to interview location number 2 plus the sampling interval, or 1858.26 + 1236.26 = 3094.52.

> **HINT:** Now go to <u>Overhead #7</u>. The location of the <u>third interview</u> will be the first community on the list with a cumulative population equal to or greater than 3094 (note: the decimal is NOT used for identifying the location).

D. Repeat this process for the <u>fourth interview</u> location, explaining that this time the number will equal interview location number 3 plus the sampling interval (3094.52 + 1236.26 = 4330.78).

E. Now ask participants to repeat this process to find the interview location (number) for the 5th, 6th, 7th, 8th, 9th, and 10th interviews.

Have them fill in the blanks that have been left for these interviews on their copy of Overhead #6. Allow <u>10 to 15 minutes</u> for this task. The trainer(s) should walk around the room checking participants' work. If necessary, use the Answer Guide for Overhead 6, but do not show it to participants until STEP 8 is finished. Record the answers on Overhead #6.

> **See answer guide for correct answers to OVERHEAD #6**

F. Display Overhead #7: LQAS Sampling Frame for a Supervision Area. Look for the first community with a cumulative population larger than the first interview location number that is the number selected from the random number table (0622). The community is Santai. Show that the number for the first interview location has already been recorded in column 4 row 2. Now show them where the second interview location number is found. Find the first community equal to or less than 1858 (Serina.) Complete column 4 in a group or have participants complete it individually. Check their work.

Explain the meaning of the three location numbers on the chart for the town of Pingra (9275, 10512, 11748).

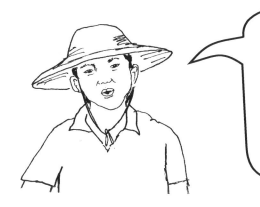

Pingra will be the location of 3 interviews (#8, #9, #10) because of its relatively large total population (3504, largest on the list), meaning that when the location number of the 8th interview (Pingra) was added to the sampling interval (1236.26) to determine the location number of the 9th interview, we still had not reached a number greater than the cumulative population of Pingra.

Module 2, Session 1

Point out how this makes sense for doing a survey because we want to go to those places where most of the people we are serving live. (If you want to be daring, don't explain this; ask, rather, if anyone in the group can give it.)

G. Finally, you can now fill in the far-right column on Overhead #7 (Number of Interviews) for the various locations, depending on the location number. The total, of course, will be 19 locations.

> **See answer guide for correct answers to OVERHEAD #7**

STEP 8—If adjustments need to be made to any of the organization's sampling frames, assign participants the job of repeating the tasks practiced in this session using their own supervision area.

> **SUGGESTION: Tell trainees that they will need to identify specific interview locations (using a random process) for the survey they will complete later in this training (if it has not been done already). Therefore, over the next two days they should review the eight steps shown in this Session with the data from their own supervision areas, and the locations for the 19 interviews. (If locations have already been selected, participants should go through the steps to confirm the location of the 19 interviews.**

Once they have chosen the 19 locations, they should then develop a travel plan (with the NGO program manager and the lead trainers) for visiting each location on the days scheduled for the survey. (State the days.) Participants should review their calculations and their travel plans with the training workshop leaders.

> **SUGGESTION: As an alternative to doing this session with supervisors, managers of each organization participating in the training can complete this task of identifying interview locations for each supervision area they are responsible for.**

Answer Guide for Overhead 6
(Note: This answer guide should not appear in the participant's manual)

Identify the Location of Each of the 19 Interviews in a Supervision Area

Random Number = 622   Sampling Interval = 1236.26

No.	Calculation	Interview Location
1.	Random Number	622
2.	RN + Sampling Interval	1858
3.	Interview Location Number 2 + Sampling Interval	3094
4.	Interview Location Number 3 + Sampling Interval	4330
5.	Interview Location Number 4 + Sampling Interval	5567
6.	Interview Location Number 5 + Sampling Interval	6803
7.	Interview Location Number 6 + Sampling Interval	8039
8.	Interview Location Number 7 + Sampling Interval	9275
9.	Interview Location Number 8 + Sampling Interval	10512
10.	Interview Location Number 9 + Sampling Interval	11748
11.	Interview Location Number 10 + Sampling Interval	12984
12.	Interview Location Number 11 + Sampling Interval	14220
13.	Interview Location Number 12 + Sampling Interval	15457
14.	Interview Location Number 13 + Sampling Interval	16693
15.	Interview Location Number 14 + Sampling Interval	17929
16.	Interview Location Number 15 + Sampling Interval	19165
17.	Interview Location Number 16 + Sampling Interval	20402
18.	Interview Location Number 17 + Sampling Interval	21638
19.	Interview Location Number 18 + Sampling Interval	22874

Answer Guide for Overhead 7
(Note: This answer guide should not appear in the participant's manual)

LQAS Sampling Frame for a Supervision Area

Name of Community	Total Population	Cumulative Population	Interview Location Number	Number of Interviews
Pagai	548	548		
Santai	730	1278	622.00	1
Serina	686	1964	1858.26	1
Mulrose	280	2244		
Fanta	1256	3500	3094.52	1
Bagia	684	4184		
Rostam	919	5103	4330.78	1
Mt. Sil	1374	6477	5567.04	1
Livton	1136	7610	6803.30	1
Farry	544	8154	8039.56	1
Tunis	193	8347		
Pulau	375	8722		
Sasarota	333	9055		
Pingra	3504	12559	9275.82, 10512.08, 11748.34	3
Kanata	336	12895		
Sirvish	2115	15010	12984.6, 14220.86	2
Balding	258	15268		
Rescuut	678	15946	15457.12	1
Krista	207	16153		
Manalopa	1162	17315	16693.38	1
Garafa	408	17723		
Spiltar	455	18178	17929.64	1
Masraf	978	19156		
Abrama	335	19491	19165.90	1
Junagadh	541	20032		
Singri	725	20757	20402.16	1
Kalarata	355	21112		
Ichimota	498	21610		
Chaplar	347	21957	21638.42	1
Sr. Kitt	186	22143		
Nevis	1346	23489	22874.68	1
TOTAL	**23489**			**19**

MODULE THREE

Whom should I interview?

Session 1: Selecting Households

Session 2: Selecting Respondents

Session 3: Field Practical for Numbering and Selecting Households

MODULE THREE/Session 1: Selecting Households

PURPOSE: Participants have identified the general locations of their 19 interviews. They now need to advance to the next step of selecting respondents and selecting the household(s) they will visit at each location.

TIME 90 minutes.

OBJECTIVES By the end of this session, participants will have:

1. Evaluated case examples of selecting households.
2. Selected a "household" at random as a starting point for a survey.

PREPARATION Before you begin this session, prepare two large maps showing houses, rivers, roads, and other landmarks.

DELIVERY **STEP 1**—Introduce this session.

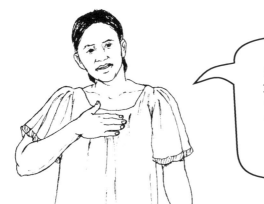

We are assuming that we have identified the locations for the 19 interviews and have now gone to the first location. Our first task is to select a household at random, and this session will teach us how to do that.

> **NOTE:** There are a variety of community/neighborhood scenarios presented in Appendix 5 that will help you plan your survey.

STEP 2—Explain how to assign numbers. Display Overhead #1: How To Assign Numbers to Households (refer participants to their copy) and briefly describe how to respond to each of the three situations presented, as suggested below.

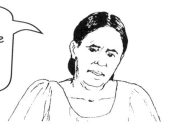

Now we need to talk about how to number the households and choose one randomly

A. The first row on the chart says: "A complete household list/map is available."

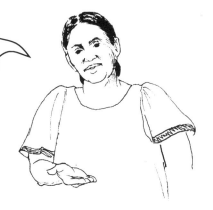

In this first situation, we have a complete household list. In this case you need only number each household on the list/map. The order of the houses is not important.

B. For the second row on the chart ("If the community size is about 30 households or fewer"), display Overhead #2: Situation 2: Household List Not Available - Size about 30.

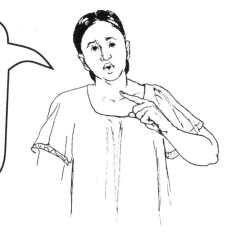

In this case the interviewer will have to draw a map of the households in that location with the help of an informant (someone who lives in the community), and then assign numbers to the houses on the completed map. If a map is available, however, review it with the informant to make sure it is accurate and then assign numbers.

Module 3, Session 1

C. For the third row ("If the community size is more than about 30 households"), display Overhead #3: Situation 3: Household List Not Available - Size more than 30. The goal is to divide a large area, with hundreds of houses, into smaller sections so we can <u>easily</u> count a few houses.

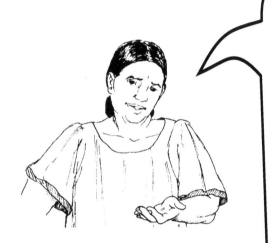

In this case, the interviewer will:

(1) learn that there are more than 30 households in the community (let's assume there are 700 households);

(2) subdivide the community into two or more equal sections;

(3) select one of these sections at random;

(4) if the selected area is still too large, subdivide it again into 2 or more equal sections, number each section, and select one section at random;

(5) continue until you have one small section with less than 15 households

(6) draw a map of the section with the help of an informant;

(7) number the households in this section on this map (you only need to count the houses in the selected section).

D. Display Overhead #4: Group of 27 Households Numbered for Random Selection of 1 Household (refer participants to their copy). Explain that now that we have numbered households in a particular location, we have to decide which houses to visit to find respondents.

E. Review selecting a random number. Explain that we need to choose a random number to select the first household and remind participants that they have already learned how to do this (using a Random Number Table) in STEP 6 of Module Two/Session 1. Ask for a volunteer to describe the process, as he/she selects a random number from a Random Number Table. In this example the number must be a two-digit number ranging from 1-27 because there are 27 houses. Remind the participants to use 2 columns only on the Random Number Table since the number 27 has 2 digits. Now find the matching house on the map.

STEP 3—Do the "Green House" exercise to show participants how to select a household to interview.

    A. <u>Have participants gather around one of the two large maps prepared earlier</u> and now displayed on a table. The map should have houses (with doors), roads, rivers, or other natural features.

    B. Now go step-by-step through the exercise described above. Pretend that no one you want to interview is at this household.

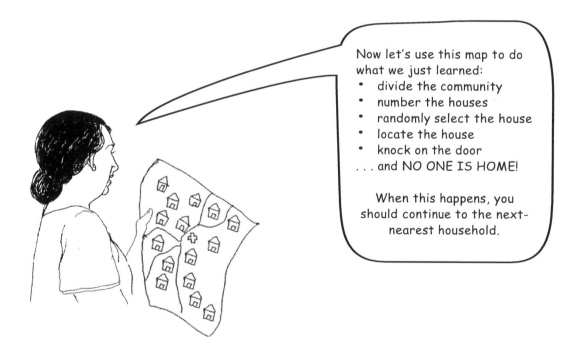

Now let's use this map to do what we just learned:
- divide the community
- number the houses
- randomly select the house
- locate the house
- knock on the door
. . . and NO ONE IS HOME!

When this happens, you should continue to the next-nearest household.

    C. Now go to the second map and <u>repeat this process</u>. To increase interest, green houses from a Monopoly game can be placed on the maps (with doors painted on one side). You could also use painted stones.

D. Explain:

> **SUGGESTION: Take participants through the process for the first four interview locations.**

STEP 4—Role-play on how to make a map in a community. Explain how to work with the community to make a map.

- A. Say, once you are in the community, find a person (an informant) who is willing to help you make a map. Often the community leader or the chief will help you, especially if you let the community know you are coming in advance.

- B. Use a page from a flip-chart to draw the map. Ask your helper to first tell you if there is a center of the community, often a plaza or a market. If there isn't a center, ask the helper to describe a place in the community where about half of the people are to the north and half to the south, or half are to the east and half are to the west.

- C. Next, have the helper draw local landmarks (churches, mosques, schools, shops, football pitches) or other well-known places. Also ask him or her where there are roads and footpaths. Draw all of these features on your map.

- D. Next, using roads and other landmarks, divide the community into 4 sections and label them 1-4. Using a random-number table, select one section randomly. Let's assume that section 3 is selected randomly.

- E. Now ask your helper to give more detail about section 3—more information about paths, roads and other landmarks. At this point he or she may want to tell you where houses are located. Draw a small box to represent each house.

- F. Now divide section 3 into 2 to 5 sub-sections that are of about the same size, using paths and other landmarks. If this is difficult to do, then go to section 3 and ask a person to take you to a place where about half the people are in front of you and half are behind you. Number the sub-sections and choose one randomly.

G. Continue until you have only a few houses remaining, few enough to easily count. Number them and choose one randomly.

H. Update your map, recording all the information collected about the community. Each time the NGO carries out a sampling in the community, they can refine the map. Since they will always choose sections and sub-sections randomly, they will almost always go to a different part of the community.

STEP 5 (Optional)— Explain the Spin-the-Bottle method. Tell participants that this method is another random way of selecting a house. However, it can be easily misused. Say that it should only be used if one of the other methods already discussed cannot be used. The simplest way to use this method is when there are a few houses (about 30) in the section of the community you have selected.
- Go to the center of that section.
- Place a bottle on the ground. Spin it so that it rotates several times.
- Once it stops, walk in a straight line in the direction the bottle is pointing. Count the number of houses along this line.
- When you come to the boundary of the community section you selected—stop. Let's assume you counted 10 houses along this line.
- Choose a random number from 1 to 10 to choose a house.

The same method can be applied in areas with many more houses, but is much more complicated. In remote areas it is difficult to use. Avoid following paths that are near to but not in the direction the bottle points.

> **IMPORTANT: If you have two or more interview locations you have to go back to Step 4.D. to identify each of the other households.**

MODULE THREE/Session 2: Selecting Respondents

PURPOSE After participants have numbered households and randomly selected them, they are ready for the last two steps of identifying respondents: selecting a household at random and selecting a suitable respondent in that household. These two activities are the focus of this session.

TIME 90 minutes.

OBJECTIVES By the end of this session, participants will have:

1. Determined whether "households" did or did not have a suitable respondent.

2. Selected the next-nearest household to the random starting household.

PREPARATION Before you begin this session, you will need to do the following:

1. Decide what age groups of respondents you have to interview. Also decide whether you need to interview men and women. Read Appendix 2 to learn more about how to decide what respondents to interview.

2. You will need to prepare the household composition scenarios used for the role-play in STEP 4 or use the scenarios already prepared (Overhead #6). If you prepare your own, they must be of two kinds:

Those which *meet* the survey criteria, and are households with people who should be sampled (see below).

Those which *do not meet* the criteria: for example, different age or gender than needed; empty house; respondent absent or far away; can't find respondent within 30 minutes of travel.

3. You will, of course, have to decide what the survey criteria are (what type of respondent you are looking for) before you can create these scenarios. In this training we will assume only one type of respondent is used.

4. Each scenario should be printed on a separate piece of paper, with a unique number written on the back, and folded so the scenario is not visible. The scenarios on Overhead #6 can be cut into strips and used for this exercise.

DELIVERY

STEP 1—Introduce the topic of selecting the respondent. Present the type or types of respondent to be interviewed in the survey. Explain that questionnaires have been prepared earlier for these types of respondents. The types of respondents depend on the health interventions. Please see Appendix 2 for a discussion of how to prepare questionnaires if you have different types of respondents.

STEP 2—Display Overhead #5: Rules for Identifying Respondents (refer participants to their copy) and briefly go through the four scenarios outlined there.

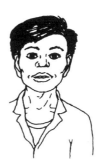

Now that we are at the house that was chosen randomly, we need to find the correct person to interview!

STEP 3—Display again Overhead #4 from Module Three/ Session 1. Show how to select a respondent.

Module 3, Session 2

> **SUGGESTION:** Go through several examples on the map in which no one that can be sampled lives in a house that has been selected. Show how it is possible to go to other locations in the community by following the rule of "going to the next nearest household from the front entrance of the household where you are." Practice going to the nearest household <u>at least 5 times</u> to show how this leads you through the community.

STEP 4—Role-play selecting respondents. Explain that now we are going to do a role-play to practice selecting respondents.

A. Divide the group into subgroups of 10-12 participants, assign a trainer to each group, and have each group move to its own part of the training area (ideally a garden).

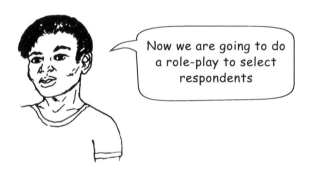

B. Give each group trainer a set of household-composition scenarios, one for each member of the group. Each scenario describes a household on one side and has a unique number on the back side (see Overhead #6).

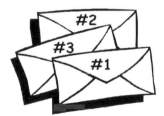

> **SUGGESTION:** Explain that each piece of paper in the envelope represents a unique household that has been assigned its own number.

C. Give a scenario to each participant and <u>arrange the participants like houses in a pretend community</u>. The direction the participant faces is the door.

D. Ask for a volunteer to select the first "household," using a random number, and then approach the person holding the scenario with that number.

> **IMPORTANT:** Each time a random number needs to be selected review how to do it using the random number table. Be sure it is clear that when selecting a 4 digit random number, the participant uses 4 columns in the table. S/he used only 2 columns when selecting 2 digit numbers.

E. Have the person holding the scenario read the description of this first household aloud and then:

> **SUGGESTION:** Ask the volunteer whether anyone in this household qualifies as the type of respondent needed. If not, what should the volunteer do? GO TO THE NEXT NEAREST HOUSE.

F. Have the volunteer move to the next nearest household or door, if necessary, until he or she finds a respondent who qualifies.

G. After the first volunteer finds a household with a suitable respondent, have other volunteers practice the steps of this process, starting with selecting a random number. Continue until most scenarios have been discussed.

> **SUGGESTION:** Entertain questions/discussion before closing the session.

MODULE THREE/Session 3: Field Practical for Numbering and Selecting Households

PURPOSE This session includes a field trip to a pre-identified community to practice numbering and selecting households.

TIME 3 hours.

OBJECTIVES By the end of this session, participants will have:

1. Assigned numbers to households to select one at random.
2. Selected a household at random as a starting point.
3. Identified the next nearest household to the starting point.

PREPARATION This session <u>needs much planning</u> and effort by the trainers. Before the start of this session, be sure to complete the following tasks:

1. Ask a trainee to identify a location that has enough sites so participants can work in groups of 10-12. Each group will need its own site of at least 40-50 households. 100-500 households also make a good, but more complex exercise.
2. Ask a trainee or a volunteer to develop a general map of the site(s).
3. Identify and meet with "gatekeepers" for each site; that is, officials and others whose permission or approval is necessary before bringing participants into the site for the training exercise. Explain to them the purpose of the exercise, ask permission to bring trainees on the scheduled days, and arrange that they or someone else can be available on those days to meet the trainees.

4. Assign participants to each of the sites (no more than 10-12 a site) and assign one facilitator to each group.
5. Arrange for transport to the sites and all other logistics.

DELIVERY

STEP 1—Introduce the session. On the day of this field practical, bring the group together to introduce this session.

> **SUGGESTION: Explain the preparations you have made and explain that the goal of this exercise is to practice numbering and selecting households in an actual site.**

STEP 2—Explain the protocol for entering the community. Have the person who arranged the field visit present the site map(s) (drawn in #2 under preparation) and explain with whom the group will meet in the community.

STEP 3—Review the steps of the field practical. Display Overhead #7: Process for Field Practical (refer participants to their copy) and discuss each of the steps. Also display and discuss the site maps developed for this exercise. Inform participants which site they have been assigned to, any arrangements that have been made for meals, and the logistics of drop-off and pick-up.

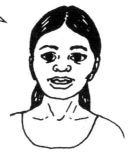

This is the process for this field practical. I would also like to tell you about the logistics for this exercise: meals, transportation, etc.

Also, if you find that once you are in your site that the map is not accurate, you will need to revise it or start again to make a new map.

Module 3, Session 3

STEP 4—Once you are at the site, take your group through the field practical using the process presented in Overhead #1.

   A. Meet with the community leader as prearranged.

   B. Create or revise the community map. Ask the community leader or someone he or she selects to corroborate the accuracy of the map you are using and make any necessary revisions.

> **IMPORTANT: If you do not have a map, walk through the community with an informant and draw one now.**

   C. If necessary, the group should now subdivide the community into multiple sections of equal size – about 2-5 sections. Number these sections and choose one at random. If the selected section is still too large an area to easily count the number of households, then continue subdividing and choosing subsections at random until you have a subsection with 15 or fewer households.

   D. The group should then number the households in the community (or in the section they have chosen) and select a starting household at random. They should select it using a random number table.

   E. Go to the first household and ask the group what they should do next.

> **Answer: Determine if an eligible respondent lives in this household.**

   F. Ask the group what they should do if a respondent of the type they are looking for does not live in this household.

> **Answer: Go to the next nearest household.**

G. Ask the group how to identify the next-nearest household.

> **Answer: It is the household closest to the front entrance of the first household selected at random.**

H. Ask the group what they would do if a respondent does not live in the next-nearest household either.

> **Answer: Go to the next nearest household.**

I. Ask the group how they would identify this household.

> **Answer: This would be the house closest to the front entrance of the house nearest the household.**

J. Ask the group what they would do if there is a suitable respondent in a household but he or she is visiting a neighbor less than 30 minutes away.

> **Answer: Ask someone to take you to him/her.**

K. Ask the group what they should do if the respondent who lives in a household is visiting a location that is far away more than 30 minutes.

> **Answer: Go to the next nearest household.**

> **NOTE:** When correctly using the "next nearest house" rule, one may move from one house to the next and cross into other sections on the community map or into other communities/villages/towns. HOWEVER, you may NEVER move into another SA.

L. Continue the process as necessary.

(The questions listed here don't have to be asked; they are more of a checklist of procedures the group should be sure to practice. The trainer, in fact, should try not to intervene in the group's work unless the group asks for help or makes a mistake.)

> **IMPORTANT:** If there are two or more interview locations in the same community, go back to Step 4.C. to identify randomly, each of the other households.

STEP 5—Debrief the field practical. After the groups finish their exercise and return to the training site (or while still in the village, if this is more suitable), lead a discussion of the experience.

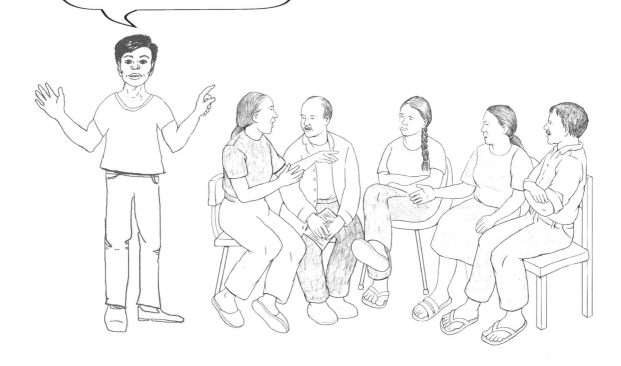

MODULE FOUR

What questions do I ask and how should I ask them?

Session 1: Reviewing the Survey Questionnaires

Session 2: Interviewing Skills

Session 3: Field Practical for Interviewing

Session 4: Planning and Doing the Data Collection/Survey

MODULE FOUR/Session 1: Reviewing the Survey Questionnaires

PURPOSE In this session, participants prepare for their survey by reviewing the questionnaires they will be using and by practicing how they will fill out these questionnaires.

TIME 1 hour *(Note: the time will vary depending on the number of questionnaires to review)*.

OBJECTIVES By the end of this session, participants will have:

1. Reviewed all the questions on the questionnaire.
2. Posed questions to clear up any confusion about the questionnaire.

PREPARATION Be sure to have the questionnaire that will be used in the survey available for this session, in more than one language if necessary. Participants will be using the questionnaire in this exercise, which will have been prepared ahead of time by the managers and other staff. This questionnaire will have been pretested in a local community similar to those where the survey will be carried out. This will ensure that most people will understand the questions and how they are phrased. Only small changes, if any, should have to be made to the questionnaire during this stage of the training.

DELIVERY **STEP 1**—Give out copies of the questionnaire and describe how it was developed.

> **SUGGESTION: Be sure to explain that this questionnaire has already been developed, modified, and pre-tested by program managers from their organizations**

STEP 2—Review the questionnaire. Go through the entire questionnaire as follows:

    A. Read through each question and make sure participants understand: (1) what information the question is asking for and (2) the purpose behind each question.

    B. Discuss all the possible responses to each question and explain what the interviewer should do in each case. Point out that some questions allow multiple responses.

    C. Explain the skip patterns in each questionnaire and what the interviewer should do in such cases.

STEP 3—Ask if there are any questions about the questionnaire. Do not make any changes to questions unless absolutely necessary. Then pretest again any questions that you change.

MODULE FOUR/Session 2: Interviewing Skills

PURPOSE The purpose of this session is to review and practice effective interviewing techniques.

TIME 1 hour and 45 minutes to 2 hours and 30 minutes.

OBJECTIVES By the end of this session, participants will have:

1. Watched a staged demonstration interview with GOOD and BAD interviewing techniques
2. Defined proper etiquette for interviewing.
3. Asked questions using good interviewing techniques.
4. Recorded answers on the questionnaire.
5. Received feedback on their interviewing skills.

PREPARATION Be sure to bring samples of the questionnaire to this session for the practice in STEP 4.

DELIVERY   **STEP 1**—Introduce the session. Display Overhead #1: Why Interviewing Is Important (refer participants to their copies) and review the key points.

In this session, by practicing interviewing using the questionnaires, participants will become familiar with them. Then, in the next session, they will have a field practice. They will be able to use the questionnaire and ask all the questions on the survey.

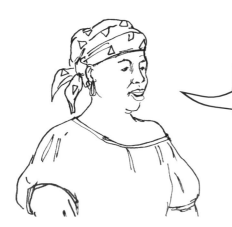

You should not be learning the questionnaire as you are interviewing people. It is important for you to <u>be familiar with the questionnaire</u> before you begin the survey. In this session we will practice working with the questionnaire.

Module 4, Session 2 69

STEP 2—Discuss interview etiquette. Display Overhead #2: Interview Etiquette and go over the key points with participants. Ask them to add any other etiquette points proper for their country or circumstances.

STEP 3—This step begins with a role-play by the trainer. One of the participants can take the role of an interviewee such as a mother of child 0-11 months of age. Using key points that are presented in Overhead #3: Effective Interviewing Techniques, carry out 2 demonstrations. Ask the participants to observe both sessions but to hold questions until both demonstrations are finished.

In the first demonstration be a **good interviewer** who uses key points listed in Overhead #3. In the second demonstration be a **poor interviewer** who violates the key points listed in Overhead #3. This session can be a lot of fun for everyone.

Now, discuss the observations and comments about both demonstrations. Lead the discussion so that the participants reveal the key points you covered in the role-plays.

Now discuss other effective interviewing techniques. Display Overhead #3: Effective Interviewing Techniques and go over each point with participants. Show them how many of techniques they discovered for themselves in the role-plays.

Be sure to spend enough time on techniques not as yet discussed. Give examples or show the techniques where suitable. Ask participants to comment and to add other points from their experience.

STEP 4—Practice interviewing. With the questionnaire to be used in the survey, have participants practice interviewing in groups of three.

A. Divide participants into groups of three.

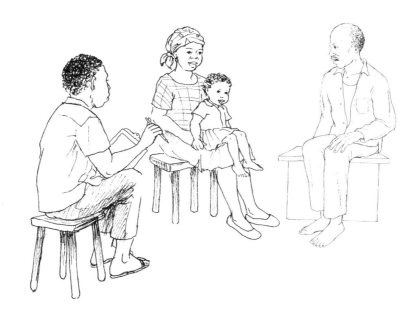

B. Have one participant play the role of the interviewer, one the role the respondent, and one an observer. The respondent will pretend he or she is the type of respondent needed for the interview. Select a questionnaire and have the interviewer ask questions of the respondent and record the answers (in pencil if you want to reuse this questionnaire in the survey or in other role-plays). The observer should make notes of any feedback he or she wants to tell the interviewer after the role-play. The observer should NOT interrupt the interviewer during the role-play.

If you think the participants need another demonstration, you can have 2 participants volunteer to do one role-play for the entire group. The trainer and other participants can jot down notes to discuss once it is over.

C. Small-group debriefing. After about 20 minutes, ask the participants to debrief the experience for about 5 minutes, with the observer and the respondent giving feedback.

D. Have the three participants conduct and debrief a second interview for another 20 minutes, changing roles so there is a different interviewer, respondent, and observer. Then have them debrief again for 5 minutes.

E. Participants change roles one last time and conduct a third interview and debriefing for 5 minutes.

> **SUGGESTION: Each member of the group will have the opportunity to be the interviewer, the respondent, and the observer if time permits.**

STEP 5—Large-group debriefing. Reconvene the entire group and lead a discussion on what went well and what could be improved.

> **SUGGESTION: Be sure to discuss strategies for avoiding or dealing with any of the common problems that arose.**

STEP 5—Encourage participants to practice more interviewing on their own before fieldwork begins. If you or the managers notice anyone having difficulty, suggest that person, his or her manager, and one other person stay behind after the session to continue to practice.

MODULE FOUR/Session 3: Field Practical for Interviewing

PURPOSE The purpose of this session is to give participants a chance to practice interviewing respondents with the questionnaire before they do their actual surveys. It is important for participants to be as familiar as possible with the survey instruments and with real interview circumstances before they conduct their own surveys. This is the time to make mistakes and become familiar with the questionnaires.

TIME 3 hours 45 minutes.

OBJECTIVES By the end of this session, each participant will have:

1. Completed <u>at least two sets of questionnaires</u> (more if possible).
2. Received a debriefing on his or her interview skills.

PREPARATION Before you begin this session, make the following preparations:

1. Like all the other field practicals, the trainers will have to lay the groundwork for this session. You will need to identify a village near the training site and get permission to come there on the appointed day to conduct interviews. Be sure there are enough households with the type of respondent needed for the exercise.
2. Make sure all the arrangements have been made to transport people to and from the site.
3. Make sure each participant brings two sets of questionnaires plus one extra as well as anything else needed to carry out the interviews. (For example pencils, pencil sharpener, eraser, clipboard, bag to carry materials, random number table, a coin to flip, raincoat.)

DELIVERY   **STEP 1**—Introduce the field practical. Explain the purpose of the exercise, the sequence of events, and any logistics.

STEP 2—Divide participants into <u>groups of no more than three</u> and assign a trainer/facilitator to each group.

STEP 3—Carry out the field practical. Transport participants to the site of the practical and continue as follows:

   A. Explain how many sets they will complete.

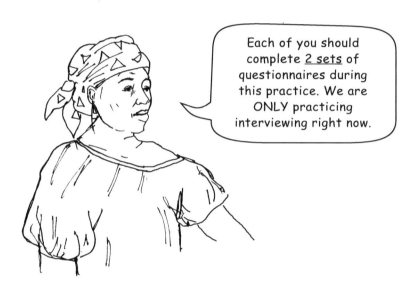

Each of you should complete <u>2 sets</u> of questionnaires during this practice. We are ONLY practicing interviewing right now.

   B. Explain the next point.

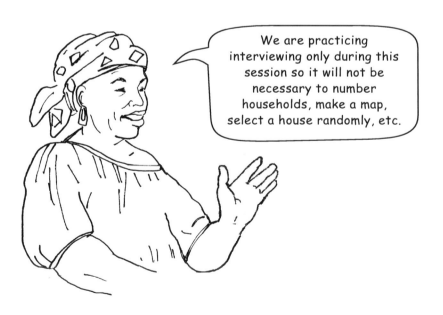

We are practicing interviewing only during this session so it will not be necessary to number households, make a map, select a house randomly, etc.

> **IMPORTANT:** It is necessary, however, that interviewers are selecting respondents properly, especially in cases where more than one person in the household fits the selection criteria. The trainers/facilitators should observe each participant in their group at least once and make notes for subsequent debriefing.

    C. Have participants carry out two interviews. Be sure each interviewer completes one interview before beginning another.

    D. Debrief participants after each interview. As suitable and possible, the trainer/facilitator debriefs his or her group members individually, away from the respondent, after the first one or two interviews. Be sure to communicate the strengths of the interviewer ("I like how you...") and areas for improvement ("How about trying...").

STEP 4—Debrief the field practical in a group. At the site or back at the training place, go over the experience, asking participants what worked well and what problems or difficulties they had. Be sure to discuss solutions for any problems that arose. Be sure that all participants agree that the people interviewed understood the questionnaires. If not, decide whether to make any changes to a questionnaire. This is your last chance! <u>But only make changes if necessary</u>. (If you change the questions, you must field-test the new questions.)

MODULE FOUR/Session 4: Planning and Doing the Data Collection/Survey

> **NOTE:** This "Session" is a set of checklists that should be taken into the field by data collectors and their managers. Each list is in the Participant's Manual. This Session contains no new material and need not be discussed by the group; if there are any questions, however, facilitators should be prepared to answer them. The lists may need to be adapted according to specifics for the survey.

PURPOSE   The purpose of this session is for interview teams to carry out the survey.

TIME   4 to 7 days per team (schedule time as needed).

OBJECTIVES   By the end of this session, each interview team will have:

1. Completed <u>19 sets of interviews with the correct type of respondents</u>.

PREPARATION   Before you begin this session, make the following preparations:

1. Make sure all the arrangements have been made to transport people to and within the project site.
2. Make sure there are 19 sets of questionnaires, PLUS 2 extra (21 sets, total) for each interview team. These should be stapled before the SA teams receive them.
3. Make sure all necessary materials are available; for example: pencils, erasers, mini stapler, random number tables, scratch paper for drawing maps. See "Materials Checklist" in the Participant's Manual for complete list of materials.

> **IMPORTANT:** During the survey phase of the training, managers, facilitators and workshop trainers should accompany participants to the field and spend the first one or two days making sure the interviews are going well and there are no other problems. Trainers and facilitators should always work through/coordinate their actions with the NGO program managers who will be in charge of this activity. Each facilitator should be assigned to an interview team for one or two days. If there are more interview teams than facilitators, teams can begin fieldwork at different times so that a facilitator can be available to accompany each one.

Remember: You can begin in any one of the selected communities and visit them in the order you prefer.

> **USE THIS MODULE TO CARRY OUT A BASELINE SURVEY OF YOUR PROGRAM**

MODULE FIVE

What do I do with the information I have collected during baseline?

Session 1: Fieldwork Debriefing

Session 2: Tabulating Results

Session 3: Analyzing Results

MODULE FIVE/Session 1: Fieldwork Debriefing

PURPOSE The purpose of this session is to bring participants together to discuss their experiences while they were collecting the baseline data. You can also find out whether there are any data missing or any other problems that you may need to address.

TIME One hour.

OBJECTIVES By the end of this session each data collector or team of collectors will have
1. Shared with each other important lessons learned during the survey.
2. Identified their needs for follow-up and planned to deal with outstanding issues.

Debriefing on these issues will be based on the following questions:

1. List what was difficult and easy about the data collection.
2. If you did not finish the data collection, what support do you need to complete it?
3. What other issues must the manager address?
4. What suggestions do you have for dealing with these issues?
5. What did you learn about your community or your project through this process?

PREPARATION
1. If necessary, have boxes available to collect and store questionnaires.
2. Also have extra copies of the questionnaires available in case there are questions you need to answer about them, or in case questionnaires become lost and need replacing.

DELIVERY

STEP 1—Have the participants report on the status of the data collection in each supervision area. Display Overhead #1: Status Report on Data Collection (refer participants to their manual) and complete the boxes for their supervision areas.

> **SUGGESTION: Discuss the manager's or team's plan to complete any outstanding interviews and tabulation.**

STEP 2—Discuss lessons learned from the data collection experience and record answers on a flip-chart. Ask participants to discuss what went well and what was difficult. For each of the difficulties, discuss suggestions for overcoming or avoiding this problem in the future.

MODULE FIVE/Session 2: Tabulating Results

PURPOSE   The main purpose of conducting a baseline survey is to find out the status of knowledge and behaviors related to specific health interventions of a project in a given area. The first step after completing a survey, therefore, is to tabulate the results from your questionnaires.

TIME   Continue until finished. The time needed will depend on the length of the questionnaire. One day, minimum, is encouraged.

OBJECTIVES   By the end of this session, participants will have:

1. Described why it's important to tabulate.
2. Tabulated the questionnaires used in the survey.
3. Used a checklist to check for errors in tabulation.

PREPARATION   This is a lengthy session which needs much preparation.

1. Participants must be told to bring their completed questionnaires to this session.
2. You will need to prepare a blank tabulation (or results) table <u>for each type of questionnaire</u> used in the survey. See STEP 2. This table must be based on the questionnaire used in the survey and, therefore, may be several pages long. You will need a copy of the blank tabulation table for each Supervision Area in the program's catchment area. See Appendix 7 for more examples.
3. The correct response key (column 3 on the tabulation table contains all the correct responses) should already be included in this tabulation table, but will be discussed with all the participants.
4. Change Overhead #2 to match a section of your blank tabulation table to be used for the demonstration.

DELIVERY   **STEP 1**—Discuss why it's important to tabulate. Explain what tabulation is:

> **IMPORTANT: TABULATION is bringing together the information collected during the interviews in a form so you can analyze it. This information is called "data."**

Then ask the group why it's important to do this. (Possible answers should be: to make program decisions; to identify priorities by SA or by program within an SA; to better assign resources.)

STEP 2—Review correct responses.

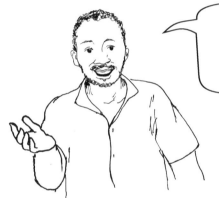

We will now review the correct responses to the questions on the questionnaire to be sure there is agreement.

Display Overhead #2: Result Tabulation Table for a Supervision Area. Show each page of the tabulation table, one at a time, to be tabulated. Cover both steps A and B below before going to the next page of the tabulation table.

> **NOTE TO TRAINER:** OVERHEAD #2 is only a SECTION of a tabulation table. We have prepared only 1 overhead in the Participant Manual to conserve space and to demonstrate the idea of the tabulation table. The actual tabulation table being reviewed in this session (which may be several pages) must be developed prior to tabulation and be based directly on the questionnaire. See Appendix 7 for more examples.

A. Read each of the questions and the correct responses already written in column 3.

> **IMPORTANT: Ask participants to stop you if they disagree and make any changes needed in the tabulation sheets to resolve any disagreements.**

B. For any question that has "skip" as a result or which may already have been skipped, discuss why the blank response equals an automatic "incorrect" or "correct." Most often an intentionally skipped response equals an "incorrect" response.

STEP 3—Show tabulation. Continue to display Overhead #2: Result Tabulation Table for a Supervision Area (or use a handout and refer participants to their copy) and lead participants through the following sequence of activities. **(Note: This manual contains only a sample table. The table must be developed from the questionnaire used during the survey.)**

A. Prepare participants for tabulation.

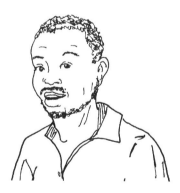

Let's begin tabulation. First, please gather all the completed questionnaires you have for one SA. The questionnaires should be ordered LQAS # 1-19. Then, for the tabulation, it is best to work in groups of 3.

In other settings there may be one long questionnaire (perhaps in modules but all together and stapled) and the tabulation table on the overhead will need to reflect one section of the long questionnaire. Therefore participants would need to flip the pages of the questionnaire to the section(s) matching the sections on the overhead's tabulation table.

B. Explain that whenever possible tabulation should be done <u>in groups of three</u>:

- The first person reads the question number and correct answers from "column 3" of the tabulation sheet.

- The second person, simultaneously, looks at the answer on the questionnaire and decides if the response on the survey is "correct" or "incorrect" and calls out the code.

- The first person then records the answer on the tabulation sheet.

- The third person corroborates that the second person correctly determined if the answer should be coded "1" or "0" or "S" or "X" and that the first person recorded it correctly. If the response was intentionally skipped, then a code of "1," "0" or "S" is possible. (See D.4.)

---

0 = incorrect answer

1 = correct answer

S = question cannot be coded 0 or 1 according to instructions on the questionnaire

X = missing response (where there should be a response)

Working in a group of three may seem tedious and unnecessary, but as tabulation progresses participants become tired and more errors will be made. The three people can change roles to share the work.
(The meaning or codes for "S" and "X" are described below in D.4.)

C. Fill in blank lines at the top of the table (such as NGO, name of SA, name of supervisor).

D. Begin tabulation with a demonstration. Organize a <u>group of three people</u>, including the trainer as one. Select one of the questions to be tabulated (one that is of particular interest to the audience) and do the following:

   1) Trainer (first person) reads the question number and answer(s) from the tabulation sheet.

2) Second person reviews the response on one questionnaire and calls out whether it is correct.
3) Trainer repeats this information.
4) If not corrected (by third person), the trainer records the information on the tabulation table:

- Write a "0" for an incorrect answer.

- Write a "1" for a correct answer.

- If a question was skipped <u>through instruction of the questionnaire</u>, then any one of three values ("0," "1," or "S") could result.

On many occasions a skipped question has the same meaning as a "0" and should be recorded as "0."

SKIPPED = "0," FOR EXAMPLE: Usually a question is skipped because the interviewee did not know the answer to a filter question (e.g., have you ever heard of HIV/AIDS); in this case all the following questions are automatically incorrect and should be recorded as "0." For example, if the respondent had never heard of HIV/AIDS, then she does not know ways to prevent HIV transmission.

On occasion, a skipped question means the same as a correct response and should be coded as "1" because it equals a correct response.

SKIPPED = "1," FOR EXAMPLE: There may be questions in which a positive response requires that subsequent questions are skipped. If we ask a respondent a question to learn if she started breastfeeding her child within the first hour of birth and she responds "Yes," then we skip the following question asking her if she fed her baby colostrum. Because she started breastfeeding her baby within one hour of birth, the skipped response is automatically correct and coded as "1."

On other occasions, a skip means the respondent should be taken out of the denominator altogether. These cases should be coded as "S."

SKIPPED = "S," FOR EXAMPLE: If a set of questions concerns the treatment of a child who has had diarrhea within the last 2 weeks, and the respondent's child has <u>not</u> had diarrhea, then those questions would not apply. In this case, write an "S" in the table. See Appendix 7 for tabulation tables designed for these types of questions.

- Write an "X" to show no response is written on the questionnaire where there should be a response (there is a missing answer). An "X" means we do not know whether the response is a "1" or a "0." Later, all the "Xs" will be removed from the analysis and from the denominator.

  There should be very few missing answers. If there are too many, then the program manager or trainer should send the interviewer back to the communities to get the missing information.

  5) Third person corroborates that the information written down is correct.

E. Repeat this process for the remaining 18 questionnaires for that question. Occasionally, the trainer should repeat or write down the "wrong" information which the second person then has to correct.

IMPORTANT: It is very important to tell participants that we are recording the responses to one question for all 19 questionnaires ONLY FOR THE PURPOSES OF THIS DEMONSTRATION. **This is to show how to make an LQAS judgement. In actual practice, it is much better to code the responses to ALL the questions on one questionnaire before going on to another questionnaire.**

F. <u>Repeat this entire process</u> for another question. Use a different volunteer and have another participant assume the recorder role.

G. After you have completed two questions (the horizontal row) for all 19 questionnaires, show filling in the two boxes at the end of each row. These are the extreme right-hand columns.

> **Total Number Correct = count all the "1"s**
>
> ** if skipped question is considered CORRECT (or equal to 1) then count it in the total correct.

1) For the column called Total Correct in SA, add up all the boxes where there is a "1" and write this number in the box.

> **Total Sample Size = count all the "1"s and "0"s**
>
> ** total should be 19 unless there is an "X" or "S" not counted as a "1" or "0."

2) For the column called Total Sample Size, add up all the boxes where there is a "1" and a "0" and write this number in the box. The total should be 19 unless there is an "X" or an "S" that was not counted as a "1" or a "0."

REMEMBER that a skipped question should always be entered as a "1" or "0" if it is equal to a "1" or a "0."

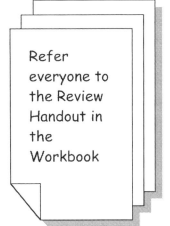

Refer everyone to the Review Handout in the Workbook

STEP 4— Review Handout: Tabulation Quality Checklist. Review each step, confirming with the participants that they understand each one. Ask them to review the checklist in their work teams and to keep doing this during the tabulation.

STEP 5— Ask participants to work in their SA teams to tabulate all the remaining questions from all questionnaires from their SA, according to the instructions in A.-E. below. While participants are doing this and all other tabulation work, the trainers should spend time with each team as they work and be sure to do the following:

Module 5, Session 2

☑ Check that teams are using the correct tabulation table and type of questionnaire.

☑ Check that teams are using an adequate procedure for calling out, recording, and verifying marks on the tabulation table.

☑ Verify all "S" and "X" codes, and review questions that should have some "S" codes to be sure participants are using the correct codes.

☑ Check that teams are using the Tabulation Quality Checklist.

☑ Answer questions that arise.

Each team will:

A. Appoint a caller, a recorder, and a verifier.

B. Go through each questionnaire one at a time, filling in the information for all questions in the tabulation sheet (in other words, move vertically down the tabulation table page). Use the procedure described under STEP 3-D above.

C. Refer to the Tabulation Quality Checklist periodically during the tabulation to be sure that they are still on track and following the procedure.

D. Stop after completing the first questionnaire on their own and ask the trainer/facilitator to <u>check the group's work before going on to the next questionnaire</u>.

E. When they have completed all questionnaires (for all questions), fill in the two columns at the far right (Total Number Correct and Total SA Sample Size) as described under STEP 3-G above.

F. If there is more than one type of questionnaire, this step will have to be carried out for them as well. Once data from one questionnaire have been entered into the tabulation table, ask SA teams to move onto the next questionnaire. Remember that each questionnaire will have its own tabulation tables.

> **NOTE: As a general rule, allow 20-30 minutes to complete a single tabulation table.**

MODULE FIVE/Session 3: Analyzing Results

PURPOSE   In this session, workshop participants will practice simple analysis of data and become familiar with a useful format for reporting data.

TIME   2 hours 15 minutes. Times vary according to the number of SAs for the organization. The number of SAs influence the time needed to complete the summary tabulation tables.

OBJECTIVES   By the end of this session, participants will have:

1. Used a summary tabulation sheet to identify low-performing SAs for each indicator.
2. Calculated average coverage.
3. Reviewed how to use an LQAS table to judge SAs.
4. Identified priorities among SAs and among indicators for the same SA using the summary results.
5. Used a useful format for reporting survey findings.

PREPARATION   Before you begin this session, you will need to do the following:

1. Prepare summary tabulation sheets in advance, based on the tabulation tables used in Module 5 Session 2.
2. Change Overhead #6: Baseline Survey Report Format used in STEP 6 to suit the needs of the project.
3. Provide calculators for participants to use.

DELIVERY

STEP 1—Show how to complete a summary tabulation sheet. Present Overhead #3: Summary Tabulation Sheet for Baseline Survey. This overhead is an example only. You should prepare in advance an example summary tabulation sheet <u>for your own program,</u> based on the questionnaire used in the survey.

Module 5, Session 3   89

A. Prepare participants for completing the summary table.

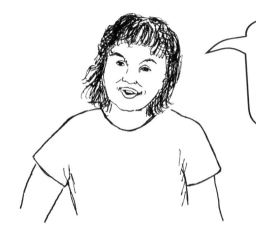

Please gather all your individual tabulation sheets and organize them by SA. For each SA we will first record the "Total SA Correct" and the "Total SA Sample Size."

B. Explain transferring information from the individual tabulation table to the summary table.

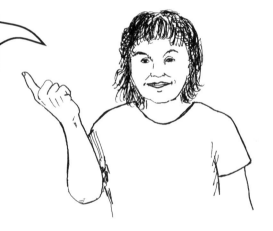

For each SA we will now transfer the "Total SA Correct" and the "Total SA Sample Size" from the individual tabulation table to the appropriately labeled columns on the summary table. This information has already been totaled and is available on the individual tabulation sheets for each SA.

C. Using an overhead, have a participant read the "Total SA Correct" and "Total SA Sample Size" for each SA for <u>one indicator</u> while the trainer records the numbers on Overhead #3.

IMPORTANT: The "Total SA Correct" is recorded above the split row.

D. Next add the total correct for all SAs together and record the results in the column "Total Correct in Program" for each indicator. Do the same for the "Total Sample Size in Program" by adding together the "Total SA Sample Sizes."

E. Calculate the "average coverage" and complete that column.

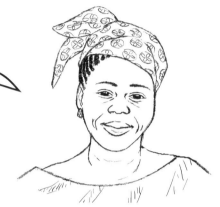

> Again, average coverage is the percentage of people in a catchment area who know of and/or practice a recommended health behavior or receive a particular service. Average coverage data are more accurate if data from at least five SAs are added together. Also, average coverage should not be computed for any indicator with data for fewer than three SAs.

STEP 2—Show how to decide which indicators in which SAs have below-average coverage. Display Overhead #4: The LQAS Table. (This is the same table that is used in Module One/Session 4.)

A. Find the average coverage on the percentage columns on this table.

> Let's say we calculate coverage to be 41%. We need to ROUND UP to the next highest percentage on the table—45%. PUT YOUR FINGER ON 45%.

B. Find the sample size for each SA in the far-left column (probably 19). But if an SA has a smaller sample size you need to use the row corresponding to that number.

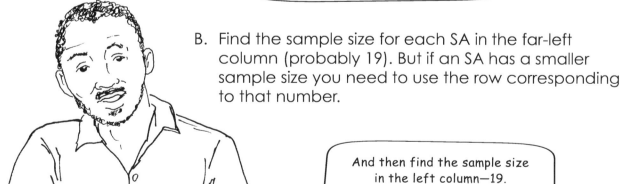

> And then find the sample size in the left column—19. PUT ANOTHER FINGER ON 19.

Module 5, Session 3

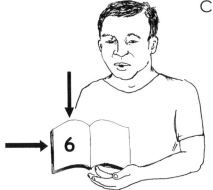

C. Bring the first finger down the page (from 45% coverage column) and the other finger across the page (from sample size 19).

> **IMPORTANT:** Where your fingers meet is the decision rule (6 in this example). However, if an SA has a sample size of 17 then the decision rule would be 5.

D. Now find and record the decision rule for all other SAs and indicators, which is <u>6 in this case</u>.

E. In the split row, record the decision rule below the total correct for the same SA (on Overhead #3). Ask participants <u>to circle indicators for any SAs that are below the decision rule</u>.

> **SUGGESTION:** Explain that these are indicators and SAs needing special attention because they have below-average coverage.

STEP 3—Explain the relation between baseline surveys and monitoring. Display Overhead #5: Defining Program Goals and Annual Targets.

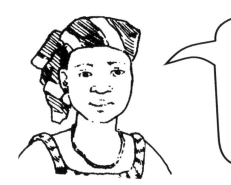

> During routine monitoring you can also use LQAS to determine whether interventions are reaching coverage targets established for a particular period. Through data collection, analysis, and planning, teams are able to adjust their program goals, refocus their resources, and maximize their achievements over time.

Display Overhead #6: Monitoring Targets and Average Coverage Over Time: In a Catchment Area. This graph compares planned annual targets to the measured annual average coverage for a catchment area. Explain that repeating data collection, analysis, and program planning in the future produces this information.

STEP 4—Have participants practice using the summary tables to analyze data and identify priorities. Ask participants to form small groups with the other members of their organization. If one organization has many participants, they can divide into subgroups based on experience or common interests (for example, safe motherhood, child health, HIV/AIDS). Then display Overhead #7: How To Analyze Data and Identify Priorities Using the Summary Tables and have each group discuss the points described on this overhead. Have overhead transparencies or flipchart paper available for participants to use to present their findings to the whole group.

STEP 5—Have participants discuss and plan average targets for the coming year.

Ask participants to select key indicators on which they want to have an impact in the next 12 months. Based on the findings of their baseline study, ask the groups to set or revise annual coverage targets for each indicator.

Have participants discuss their recommendations. This discussion could be very important for the program.

STEP 6—Have participants prepare their reports.

A. Display Overhead #8: Baseline Survey Report Format and review each section heading and page limit. This format should be adapted earlier to suit the needs of the project.

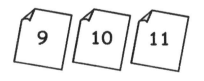

B. Display Overheads #9: Methodology, #10: Main Findings, and #11: Action Plans/Goals/Coverage targets to provide more detail for these three sections of the report.

> SUGGESTION: Ask participants to include established annual coverage targets for the coming year in their reports.

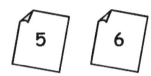

C. Display Overhead #5 and #6 again and review the program monitoring cycle and program goals/coverage targets.

D. Give participants a reasonable deadline to submit their reports—with annual coverage targets, project goals, and a time for the next monitoring of their program with LQAS.

E. You may need to visit participants one or more times while they prepare their reports and redesign their programs. They may need to review with you again how to analyze their results and decide on their priorities. This last step may be the most important step of your entire work.

You have now finished this part of the LQAS training. But your work has just begun! You should use LQAS regularly to track how well your program is progressing and make program changes when you find it is necessary to do so. LQAS will help you do that.

REMEMBER, take enough time to analyze results and plan your program. You have invested effort in collecting very good quality information. Use it well and you will improve the health conditions in the communities where you work!

> **USE THIS MODULE FOR REGULAR MONITORING OF YOUR PROGRAM**

MODULE SIX

What do I do with the information I have collected during monitoring?

Session 1: Fieldwork Debriefing

Session 2: Tabulating Results

Session 3: Analyzing Results

MODULE SIX/Session 1: Fieldwork Debriefing

PURPOSE The purpose of this session is to bring participants together to discuss their experiences while they were collecting the monitoring data. You can also find out whether there are any data missing or any other problems that you may need to address.

TIME One hour.

OBJECTIVES By the end of this session each data collector or team of collectors will have
1. Shared important lessons learned during the survey with one another.
2. Identified their needs for follow-up and planned to deal with outstanding issues.

Debriefing on these issues will be based on the following questions:

1. List what was difficult and easy about the data collection.
2. If you did not finish the data collection, what support do you need to complete it?
3. What other issues must the manager address?
4. What suggestions do you have for dealing with these issues?
5. What did you learn about your community or your project through this process?

PREPARATION
1. If necessary, have boxes available to collect and store questionnaires.
2. Also have extra copies of the questionnaires available in case there are questions you need to answer about them, or in case questionnaires become lost and need replacing.
3. Have results from baseline or previous surveys to discuss progress.

DELIVERY

STEP 1—Have the participants report on the status of the data collection in each supervision area. Display Overhead #1: Status Report on Data Collection (refer participants to their manual) and complete the boxes for their supervision area.

> **SUGGESTION: Discuss the manager's or team's plan to complete any outstanding interviews and tabulation.**

STEP 2—Discuss lessons learned from the data collection experience and record answers on a flip-chart. Ask participants to discuss what went well and what was difficult. For each of the difficulties, discuss suggestions for overcoming or avoiding this problem in the future.

MODULE SIX/Session 2: Tabulating Results

PURPOSE The main purpose of conducting a survey (except for baseline surveys) is to find out how the various health interventions in a given area are performing and as a result to be able to identify the best places (locations or specific interventions within the same location) to concentrate your resources. The first step after completing a survey, therefore, is to tabulate the results from your questionnaires.

TIME Continue until finished. The time needed will depend on the length of the questionnaire. One day, minimum, is encouraged.

OBJECTIVES By the end of this session, participants will have:

1. Described why it's important to tabulate.
2. Tabulated the questionnaires used in the survey.
3. Used a checklist to check for errors in tabulation.

PREPARATION This is a lengthy session which needs much preparation.

1. Participants must be told to bring their completed questionnaires to this session.
2. You will need to prepare a blank tabulation (or results) table <u>for each type of questionnaire</u> used in the survey. See STEP 2. This table must be based on the questionnaire used in the survey and, therefore, may be several pages long. See Appendix 7 for more examples.
3. The correct response key (column 3 on the tabulation table contains all the correct responses) should already be included in this tabulation table, but will be discussed with all the participants.
4. Change Overhead #2 to match a section of your blank tabulation table to be used for the demonstration.

DELIVERY **STEP 1**—Discuss why it's important to tabulate. Explain what tabulation is:

> **IMPORTANT: TABULATION** is bringing together the information collected during the interviews in a form so you can analyze it. This information is called "data."

Then ask the group why it's important to do this. (Possible answers should be: to make program decisions; to identify priorities by SA or by program within an SA; to better assign resources.)

If the participants have carried out LQAS several times in the past, you may be able to skip Step 1.

STEP 2—Review correct responses.

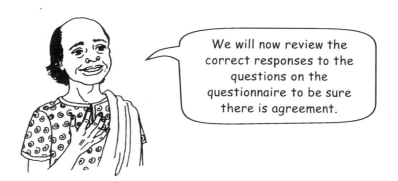

We will now review the correct responses to the questions on the questionnaire to be sure there is agreement.

Display Overhead #2: Result Tabulation Table for a Supervision Area. Show each page of the tabulation table, one at a time, to be tabulated. Cover both steps A and B below before going to the next page of the tabulation table.

> **NOTE TO TRAINER:** OVERHEAD #2 is only a SECTION of a tabulation table. We have prepared only 1 overhead in the Participant Manual to conserve space and to demonstrate the idea of the tabulation table. The actual tabulation table being reviewed in this session (which may be several pages) must be developed prior to tabulation and be based directly on the questionnaire. See Appendix 7 for more examples.

A. Read each of the questions and the correct responses already written in column 3.

> **IMPORTANT: Ask participants to stop you if they disagree and make any changes needed in the tabulation sheets to resolve any disagreements.**

B. For any question that has "skip" as a result or which may already have been skipped, discuss why the blank response equals an automatic "incorrect" or "correct." Most often an intentionally skipped response equals an "incorrect" response.

STEP 3—Show tabulation. Continue to display Overhead #2: Result Tabulation Table for a Supervision Area (or use a handout and refer participants to their copy) and lead participants through the following. **(Note: This manual contains only a sample table. The table you use must be developed from the questionnaire used during the survey.)**

A. Prepare participants for tabulation.

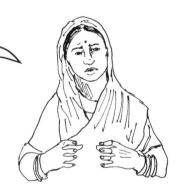

Let's begin tabulation. First, please gather all the completed questionnaires you have for one SA. The questionnaires should be ordered LQAS # 1-19. Then, for the tabulation, it is best to work in groups of 3.

Sometimes there may be one long questionnaire (perhaps in modules but all together and stapled) and the tabulation table on the overhead will need to reflect one section of the long questionnaire. Therefore participants would need to flip the pages of the questionnaire to the section(s) matching the sections on the overhead's tabulation table.

B. Explain that whenever possible tabulation should be done <u>in groups of three</u>:

- The first person reads the question number and correct answers from "column 3" of the tabulation sheet.

- The second person, simultaneously, looks at the answer on the questionnaire and decides if the response on the survey is "correct" or "incorrect" and calls out the code.

- The first person then records the answer on the tabulation sheet.

- The third person corroborates that the second person correctly determined if the answer should be coded "1" or "0" or "S" or "X" and that the first person recorded it correctly. If the response was intentionally skipped, then a code of "1," "0" or "S" is possible. (See D.4.)

Working in a group of three may seem tedious and unnecessary, but as tabulation progresses participants become tired and more errors will be made. The three people can change roles to share the work.
(The meaning or codes for "S" and "X" are described below in D.4.)

C. Fill in blank lines at the top of the table (such as NGO, name of SA, name of supervisor).

D. Begin tabulation with a demonstration using Overhead #2. Organize a <u>group of three people</u>, including the trainer as one. Select one of the questions to be tabulated (one that is of particular interest to the audience) and do the following:

   1) Trainer (first person) reads the question number and answer(s) from the tabulation sheet.

> 0 = incorrect answer
>
> 1 = correct answer
>
> S = question cannot be coded 0 or 1 according to instructions on the questionnaire
>
> X = missing response (where there should be a response)

2) Second person reviews the response on one questionnaire and calls out whether it is correct.
3) Trainer repeats this information.
4) If not corrected (by third person), the trainer records the information on the tabulation table as shown in Overhead #2:

- Write a "0" for an incorrect answer.

- Write a "1" for a correct answer.

- If a question was skipped <u>through instruction of the questionnaire</u>, then any one of three values ("0," "1," or "S") could result.

On many occasions a skipped question has the same meaning as a "0" and should be recorded as "0."

> SKIPPED = "0," FOR EXAMPLE: Usually a question is skipped because the interviewee did not know the answer to a filter question (e.g., have you ever heard of HIV/AIDS); in this case all the following questions are automatically incorrect and should be recorded as "0." For example, if the respondent had never heard of HIV/AIDS, then she does not know ways to prevent HIV transmission.

On occasion, a skipped question means the same as a correct response and should be coded as "1" because it equals a correct response.

> SKIPPED = "1," FOR EXAMPLE: There may be questions in which a positive response requires that subsequent questions are skipped. If we ask a respondent a question to learn if she started breastfeeding her child within the first hour of birth and she responds "Yes," then we skip the following question asking her if she fed her baby colostrum. Because she started breastfeeding her baby within one hour of birth, the skipped response is automatically correct and coded as "1."

On other occasions, a skip means the respondent should be taken out of the denominator altogether. These cases should be coded as "S."

SKIPPED = "S," FOR EXAMPLE: If a set of questions concern a child who has had diarrhea within the last 2 weeks, and the respondent's child has <u>not</u> had diarrhea, then those questions would not apply. In this case, write an "S" in the table. See Appendix 7 for tabulation tables designed for these types of questions.

- Write an "X" to show no response is written on the questionnaire where there should be a response (there is a missing answer). An "X" means we do not know whether the response is a "1" or a "0." Later, all the "Xs" will be removed from the analysis and from the denominator.

    There should be very few missing answers. If there are too many, then the program manager or trainer should send the interviewer back to the communities to get the missing information.

    5) Third person corroborates that the information written down is correct.

E. Repeat this process for the remaining 18 questionnaires for that question. Occasionally, the trainer should repeat or write down the "wrong" information which the second person then has to correct.

IMPORTANT: It is very important to tell participants that we are recording the responses to one question for all 19 questionnaires ONLY FOR THE PURPOSES OF THIS DEMONSTRATION. This is to show how to make an LQAS decision. In actual practice, it is much better to code the responses to ALL the questions on one questionnaire before going on to another questionnaire.

Total Number Correct = count all the "1"s

** if skipped question is considered CORRECT (or equal to 1) then count it in the total correct.

Total Sample Size = count all the "1"s and "0"s

** total should be 19 unless there is an "X" or "S" not counted as a "1" or "0."

Refer everyone to the Review Handout in the Workbook

F. <u>Repeat this entire process</u> for another question. Use a different volunteer and have another participant assume the recorder role.

G. After you have completed two questions (the horizontal row) for all 19 questionnaires, show how to fill in the two boxes at the end of each row. These are the extreme right-hand columns.

  1) For the column called Total Correct in SA, add up all the boxes where there is a "1" and write this number in the box.

  2) For the column called Total Sample Size, add up all the boxes where there is a "1" and a "0" and write this number in the box. The total should be 19 unless there is an "X" or an "S" that was not counted as a "1" or a "0."

  REMEMBER that a skipped question should always be entered as a "1" or "0" if it is equal to a "1" or a "0."

STEP 4— Review Handout: Tabulation Quality Checklist. Review each step, confirming with the participants that they understand each one. Ask them to review the checklist in their work teams and to keep doing this during the tabulation.

STEP 5— Ask participants to work together to tabulate all the remaining questions from all questionnaires from their SA, according to the instructions in A.-F. below. While participants are doing this and all other tabulation work, the trainers should spend time with each team as they work and be sure to do the following:

☑ Check that teams are using the correct tabulation table and type of questionnaire.

☑ Check that teams are using an adequate procedure for calling out, recording, and verifying marks on the tabulation table.

☑ Verify all "S" and "X" codes, and review questions that should have some "S" codes to be sure participants are using the correct codes.

☑ Check that teams are using the Tabulation Quality Checklist.

☑ Answer questions that arise.

Each team will:

A. Appoint a caller, a recorder, and a verifier.

B. Go through each questionnaire one at a time, filling in the information for all questions in the tabulation sheet (in other words, move vertically down the tabulation table page). Use the procedure described under STEP 3-D above.

C. Refer to the Tabulation Quality Checklist periodically during the tabulation to be sure that they are still on track and following the procedure.

D. Stop after completing the first questionnaire on their own and ask the trainer/facilitator to <u>check the group's work before going on to the next questionnaire</u>.

E. Ask them to fill in the two columns at the far right (Total Number Correct and Total SA Sample Size) as described under STEP 3-G above.

F. If there is more than one type of questionnaire, this step will have to be carried out for them as well. Once data from one questionnaire have been entered into the tabulation table, ask SA teams to move on to the next questionnaire. Remember that each questionnaire will have its own tabulation tables.

> **NOTE: As a general rule, allow 20-30 minutes to complete a single tabulation table.**

Module 6, Session 2   **105**

MODULE SIX/Session 3: Analyzing Results

PURPOSE — In this session, workshop participants will practice simple analysis of data and become familiar with a useful format for reporting data.

TIME — 2 hours 15 minutes. Times vary according to the number of SAs for the organization. The number of SAs influence the time needed to complete the summary tabulation tables.

OBJECTIVES — By the end of this session, participants will have:

1. Used a summary tabulation sheet to identify low-performing SAs for each indicator.
2. Calculated average coverage.
3. Reviewed how to use an LQAS table to judge SAs.
4. Identified priorities among SAs and among indicators for the same SA using the summary results.
5. Used a useful format for reporting survey findings.

PREPARATION — Before you begin this session, you will need to do the following:

1. Prepare summary tabulation sheets in advance, based on the tabulation tables used in Module 6 Session 2.
2. Change Overhead #8: Monitoring Survey Report Format used in STEP 6 to suit the needs of the project.
3. Provide calculators for the use of participants.
4. Ask the managers to bring the coverage targets they already set for each indicator.

DELIVERY

STEP 1—Show how to complete a summary tabulation sheet. Present Overhead #3: Summary Tabulation Sheet for Regular Monitoring. This overhead is an example only. You should prepare in advance an example summary tabulation sheet <u>for your own program,</u> based on the questionnaire used in the survey.

A. Prepare participants for completing the summary table.

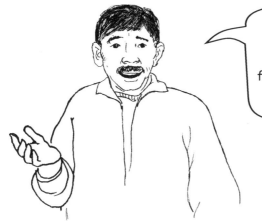

Please gather all your individual tabulation sheets and organize them by SA. For each SA we will first record the "Total SA Correct" and the "Total SA Sample Size."

B. Explain transferring information from the individual tabulation table to the summary table.

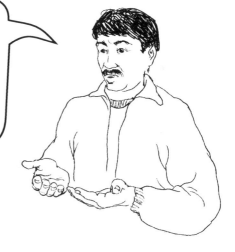

For each SA we will now transfer the "Total SA Correct" and the "Total SA Sample Size" from the individual tabulation table to the appropriately labeled columns on the summary table. This information has already been totaled and is available on the individual tabulation sheets for each SA.

C. Using an overhead, have a participant read the "Total SA Correct" and "Total SA Sample Size" for each SA for <u>one indicator</u> while the trainer records the numbers on Overhead #3.

IMPORTANT: The "Total SA Correct" is recorded above the split row.

D. Next add the total correct for all SAs together and record the results in the column "Total Correct in Program" for each indicator. Do the same for the "Total Sample Size in Program" by adding together the "Total SA Sample Sizes."

E. Calculate the "average coverage" and complete that column.

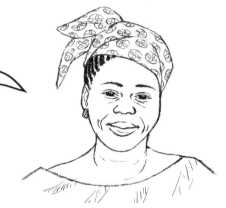

Again, average coverage is the percentage of people in a catchment area who know of and/or practice a recommended health behavior or receive a particular service. Average coverage data are more accurate if data from at least five SAs are added together. Also, average coverage should not be computed for any indicator with data for fewer than three SAs.

STEP 2—Show how to decide which indicators in which SAs have below-average coverage. Display Overhead #4: The LQAS Table. (This is the same table that is used in Module One/Session 4.)

A. Find the average coverage on the percentage columns on this table.

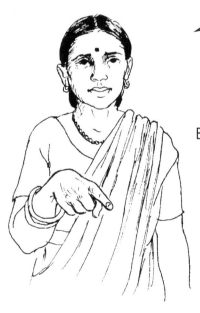

Let's say we calculate coverage to be 41%. We need to ROUND UP to the next highest percentage on the table—45%. PUT YOUR FINGER ON 45%.

B. Find the sample size for each SA in the far-left column (probably 19). But if an SA has a smaller sample size you need to use the row corresponding to that number.

And then find the sample size in the left column—19. PUT ANOTHER FINGER ON 19.

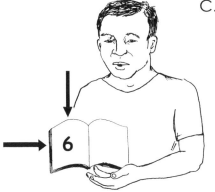

C. Bring the first finger down the page (from 45% coverage column) and the other finger across the page (from sample size 19).

> **IMPORTANT:** Where your fingers meet is the decision rule (6 in this example). However, if an SA has a sample size of 17 then the decision rule would be 5.

D. Now find and record the decision rule for all other SAs and indicators, which is <u>6 in this case</u>.

E. Record in the left cell below each split row the decision rule below the total correct for the matching SA (on Overhead #3). Ask participants <u>to circle indicators for any SAs that are below the decision rule</u>.

> **SUGGESTION:** Explain that these are indicators and SAs needing attention because they have below-average coverage.

STEP 3—Show how to decide whether interventions are reaching <u>coverage targets</u>. Display Overhead #5: Defining Program Goals and Annual Targets.

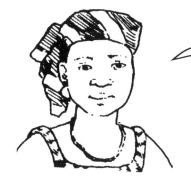

> During routine monitoring you can also use LQAS to determine whether interventions are reaching coverage targets established for a particular period.

Again, display Overhead #3: Summary Tabulation Sheet for Regular Monitoring. Point to the last column of the summary table marked "Coverage Target." Have them write the coverage target for each indicator in the space provided.

Review with the participants the current performance targets, which have been discussed and set by program managers and their teams. If the program does not have annual targets, the participants should calculate the average coverage and identify SAs that fall below it.

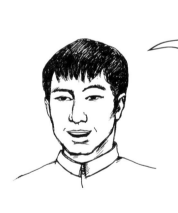

A. Display Overhead #4 again (the LQAS Table). Find the coverage target on the percentage columns on this table. Let's assume an annual coverage target of 50% for women (15-49 years) who know two or more ways to prevent HIV transmission. Ask participants to find the column labeled 50% and put a finger there.

B. Find the sample size for an SA (19) in the far left column and put another finger there.

C. Bring the fingers together to find the decision rule (where the fingers converge), which is <u>7 in this case</u>.

D. Have them write the coverage target decision rule next to and at the right of the decision rule you already entered for average coverage.

> Please mark the indicators that are below the decision rule with a star (*).

> ... These are indicators and SAs needing special attention because they are below the 50% performance coverage target.

See answer guide for correct answers to OVERHEAD #1

E. Display Overhead #6: How to Identify Priority SAs During Regular Monitoring. Tell participants that they can find the highest-priority SA among those already circled because they did not reach a coverage target or because they are below average (as already discussed earlier in STEP 2). Do so in the following manner:

1) Display Overhead #7: Using LQAS to Assess One Indicator. If an SA is circled because it is below average <u>and</u> is marked with a star (*) because it has not reached the coverage target, it is the <u>highest-priority SA</u>.

IMPORTANT: SAs with <u>both a circle and a star</u> have the lowest coverage of all since they are both below the annual coverage target and below average.

---

2) If the SA is marked with only a star (*) or a circle, then it is the next-highest priority.

3) Display Overhead #8: Monitoring Targets and Average Coverage Over Time: In a Catchment Area. This overhead is a graphical representation of Overhead #7 and can be used to reinforce the idea of monitoring a project's goals and progress at different time points—such as each year. It compares planned annual targets to the measured annual coverage for a catchment area.

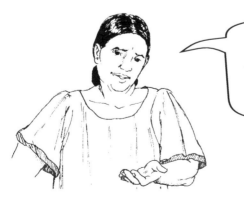

Through repeated data collection, analysis, and planning, teams are able to adjust their program goals, refocus their resources, and maximize their achievements over time.

Module 6, Session 3

STEP 4—Have participants practice using the summary tables to analyze data and identify priorities. Then display Overhead #9: How To Analyze Data and Identify Priorities Using the Summary Tables. Have overhead transparencies or flip-chart paper available for participants to use to present their findings to the whole group.

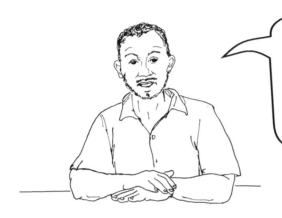

Please form small groups with the other members of your organoization and discuss the points on Overhead #9. If there are many participants, you can divide into subgroups based on experience or common interests (safe motherhood, child health, HIV/AIDS, etc.).

STEP 5—Have participants discuss and plan average targets for the coming year.

Ask participants to select key indicators on which they want to have an impact in the next 12 months. Based on the findings of their monitoring study, ask the groups to set or revise annual coverage targets for each indicator.

Have participants discuss their recommendations. This discussion could be very important for the program.

STEP 6—Have participants prepare their reports.

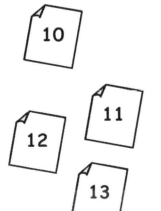

A. Display Overhead #10: Monitoring Survey Report Format and review each section heading and page limit. This format should be changed earlier to suit the needs of the project.

B. Display Overheads #11: Methodology, #12: Main Findings, and #13: Action Plans/Goals/Coverage targets to provide more detail for these three sections of the report.

> **SUGGESTION: Ask participants to include established annual coverage targets for the coming year in their reports.**

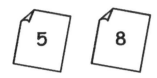

C. Display Overhead #5 and #8 again and review the program monitoring cycle and program goals/coverage targets.

D. Give participants a reasonable deadline to submit their reports, with revised annual coverage targets, project goals, and a time for the next monitoring of their program with LQAS.

E. You may need to visit participants one or more times while they prepare their reports and redesign their programs. They may need to review with you again how to analyze their results and decide on their priorities. This last step may be the most important step of your entire work.

You have now finished this next part of the LQAS training. Now continue to improve your programs by learning what is working well to help you improve what is not working yet. Continue to use LQAS regularly to track how well your program is progressing and always make program changes when necessary to do so. LQAS will help you do that. Always revise your targets so you can continue improving the quality of your work.

REMEMBER, take enough time to analyze results and revise and improve your program. You have invested effort in collecting very good quality information. Use it well and you will improve the health conditions in the communities where you work!

Answer Guide for Overhead 3
(Note: This answer guide should not appear in the participant's manual)

Summary Tabulation Table: Monitoring Females 15 – 49 Years

NGO name: _____ DATE: _____

#	Indicator	Total Correct in Each SA/Decision Rule							Total Correct in Program	Sample Size						Total Sample Size in Program	Average Coverage = Total Correct Sample Size	Coverage Target
		1	2	3	4	5	6			1	2	3	4	5	6			
CIRCLE IF BELOW AVERAGE COVERAGE DECISION RULE									**MARK WITH A STAR (*) IF BELOW COVERAGE TARGET DECISION RULE**									
Section 3: Family Planning																		
1	Age of mother at first birth	13	6*	9	11	(5*)	(5*)		49	19	19	17	19	19	19	112	43.75%	50%
		6|7	6|7	5|6	6|7	6|7	6|7											
2	How long should a female wait after the birth of a child to have another?																		
3	What can a female or male do to avoid pregnancy?																		
Section 4: HIV/AIDS and Other Sexually Transmitted Infections																		
1	Have you ever heard of an illness called HIV/AIDS?																		
2	Is there anything a man can do to avoid getting HIV/AIDS?																		
3	What can a man do to avoid getting HIV/AIDS?																		
4	Is there anything a woman can do to avoid getting HIV/AIDS?																		
5	What can a woman do to avoid getting HIV/AIDS?																		

APPENDICES

Appendix 1: Sample Workshop Agenda — **Page A-2**

Appendix 2: Dealing with More Than One Respondent Type— Parallel Sampling — **Page A-9**
- Identifying Interviewees
- Interviewing Subgroups of Interviewees
- Parallel Sampling and Developing a Questionnaire
- How to Parallel Sample

Appendix 3: LQAS Table with Alpha and Beta Errors n=19 — **Page A-13**
- What Is an Alpha and Beta Error?
- Why Use a Sample of 19?

Appendix 4: Additional Random Number Tables — **Page A-16**

Appendix 5: Alternative Neighborhood/Community Scenarios — **Page A-19**

Appendix 6: How to Calculate Weighted Coverage and Confidence Intervals — **Page A-23**
- Calculating Weighted Coverage Proportions With a Confidence Interval by Hand
- Calculating Weighted Coverage Proportions with a Confidence Interval with a Computer
- How Many SAs Should I Have?

Appendix 7: Example Tabulation Tables for Sub-Samples in which You Use Aggregate Measures Only — **Page A-29**
- Results Table Exclusive Breastfeeding
- Results Table Diarrhea Prevalence and Case Management
- Summary Table Exclusive Breastfeeding
- Summary Table Diarrhea Prevalence and Case Management

Appendix 1: Example of a Detailed Agenda for Modules 1-4 Sampling and Data Collection Workshop

Day 1

Time	Module and Session	Topic	Responsible
8:00 – 8:15 a.m.	M1/S1	Opening of Workshop	
8:15 – 8:45 a.m.	M1/S1	Participant Introduction	
8:45 – 9:00 a.m.	M1/S1	Administrative and Logistical Arrangements	
9:00 – 9:30 a.m.	M1/S1	Purpose & Agenda: Skills to be Learned	
9:30 – 9:45 a.m.		Coffee/Tea Break	
9:45 –10:30 a.m.	M1/S2	Uses of Surveys	
10:30 – 11:15 a.m.	M1/S3	Random Sampling	
11:15 – 12:15 p.m.	M1/S4	Using LQAS Sampling for Surveys: • Usefulness of 19 as a Sample Size • LQAS Sampling Exercise • What a Sample of 19 Can and Cannot Do	
12:15 – 1:15 p.m.		Lunch	
1:15 – 2:00 p.m.	M1/S4	Using LQAS for Baseline Surveys:	
2:00 – 3:15 p.m.	M2/S1	Identifying Interview Locations: • Process for Selecting Locations of Interviews • How to Calculate the Cumulative Population • How to Calculate the Sampling Interval • How to Choose a Random Number • How to Use a Random Number and Sampling Interval to Identify Locations of 19 Interviews	
3:15 – 3:30 p.m.		Coffee/Tea Break	
3:30 – 5:00 p.m.	M3/S1	Selecting Households: • Importance of Updating Maps • Process for Numbering/Choosing Households • House Selection Exercises • Examples of Numbering/Choosing Households: The Green House Exercise • Learning Experience	

Day 2

Time	Module and Session	Topic	Responsible
8:00 – 9:30 a.m.	M3/S2	Selecting Informants in a Household: • Selecting the Starting Household • Identifying Informants • Role-Play for Selecting Informants: The Garden Exercise	
9:30 – 9:45 a.m.		Coffee/Tea Break	

Day 2 (continued)

Time	Module and Session	Topic	Responsible
9:45 – 12:30 p.m.	M3/S3	Field Practical for Numbering & Selecting Households • Reviewing the Field Practical • Doing the Field Practical	
12:30 – 1:30 p.m.		• Return to Workshop Site for Lunch	
1:30 – 2:15 p.m.	M3/S3	• Review of Field Practical Sampling and Lessons Learned	
2:15 – 3:45 p.m.	M4/S1	• Reviewing the Survey Questionnaires	
3:45 – 4:00 p.m.		• Tea Break	
4:00 – 5:00 p.m.	M4/S1	• Continue Reviewing Survey Questionnaires	

Day 3

Time	Module and Session	Topic	Responsible
8:00 – 9:30 a.m.	M4/S1	• Continue Reviewing Survey Questionnaires	
9:30 – 9:45 a.m.		• Coffee/Tea Break	
9:45 – 12:30 p.m.	M4/S2	• Interviewing Techniques • Role-Play with Survey Form	
12:30 – 1:15 p.m.		• Lunch	
1:15 – 5:00 p.m.	M4/S3	• Field Practical for Interviewing	

Day 4

Time	Module and Session	Topic	Responsible
8:00 – 9:30 a.m.	M4/S3	• Review of Field Practical for Interviewing and Lessons Learned	
9:30 – 9:45 a.m.		• Coffee/Tea Break	
9:45 – 11:45 a.m.	M4/S3	• Improving Interview Technique Using Role-Plays – If Needed	
11:45 – 12:30 p.m.	M4/S4	• Develop Final Plan For the Data Collection/Survey	
12:30 – 1:30 p.m.		• Lunch	
1:30 – 2:30 p.m.	M4/S4	• Develop Final Plan for Data Collection	
2:30 – 3:00 p.m.		• Workshop Certificates Awarded & Closing	

Conduct Survey: AS LONG AS IT TAKES

Sample Agenda Module 5 (Baseline Surveys): Tabulation and Data Analysis Workshop

Day 1

Time	Module and Session	Topic	Responsible
8:00 – 8:15 a.m.		Opening: Welcome Back	
8:15 – 8:30 a.m.		New Participant Introduction/Logistical Arrangements	
8:30 – 8:50 a.m.		Reviewing the Agenda for the Tabulation Workshop	
8:50 – 9:00 a.m.		Reviewing the Training Flow Chart	
9:00 – 9:30 a.m.	M5/S1	Fieldwork Debriefing • Number of SAs in Which 19 Sets of Interviews Have Been Completed • Number of SAs with Data Collection Remaining – if Any • Confirmation that All Completed Sets of Questionnaires Have Been Brought to the Workshop • Contingency Plan for Finishing Tabulation of Remaining Questionnaires	
9:30 – 9:45 a.m.		• Tea/Coffee Break	
9:45 – 10:15 a.m.	M5/S1	• Lesson Learned During Data Collection: What Went Well and What Was Challenging	
10:15 – 11:15 a.m.	M5/S2	• Agreement on Correct Answers to the Questionnaires	
11:15 – 11:20 a.m.		Purpose of Tabulation	
11:20 – 12:00 p.m.	M5/S2	How to Use the Tabulation Tables: Reviewing the • SA Results Table • Variables Not Included in the Tabulation Tables (Filter Questions)	
12:00 – 1:00 p.m.		Lunch	
1:30 – 2:30 p.m.	M5/S2	Two Exercises: Using the Tabulation Tables to • Enter Results for One Indicator in Each SA • Reviewing the Work of Each NGO • Repeating the Above Steps with A Second Indicator	

Day 1 (continued)

Time	Module and Session	Topic	Responsible
2:30 – 3:45 p.m.	M5/S2	**Tabulation Starts In Stages** • Completing the SA Results Table for Women	
3:45 – 4:00 p.m.		Tea/Coffee Break	
4:00 – 5:00 p.m.	M5/S2	Continue Tabulation in Stages	

Day 2

Time	Module and Session	Topic	Responsible
8:00 – 9:45 a.m.	M5/S2	Continue Tabulation in Stages	
9:45 – 10:00 a.m.		Tea/Coffee Break	
10:00 –12:00 p.m.	M5/S2	Continue Tabulation in Stages	
12:00 – 1:00 p.m.		Lunch	
1:00 – 5:00 p.m.	M5/S2	Continue Tabulation in Stages	

Day 3

Time	Module and Session	Topic	Responsible
8:00 – 9:45 a.m.	M5/S2	Continue Tabulation in Stages	
9:45 – 10:00 a.m.		Tea/Coffee Break	
10:00 – 12:00 p.m.	M5/S2	Continue Tabulation in Stages	
12:00 – 1:00 p.m.		Lunch	
1:00 – 2:30 p.m.	M5/S3	How to Analyze LQAS Data and Identify Priorities: • Summary Table • How to Calculate Average Coverage and Why it is Important • Identifying SAs that Are Average, Above Average from Those that Are Below the Average for Women • Priorities Within an Individual SA When Considering Several Indicators • Priorities Among Several SAs When Considering One Indicator	

Day 3 (continued)

Time	Module and Session	Topic	Responsible
2:30 – 3:00 p.m.	M5/S3	Analyzing data (cont.) and Preparing a Baseline Survey Report: • Purpose • Basic Outline: Data Analysis and Program. Planning Implications Setting Annual Goals	
3:00 – 3:15 p.m.		Tea/Coffee Break	
3:15 – 4:15 p.m.	Not in this training manual	Planning Next Steps: • Archiving Data in a Computer Data Based Project-Wide Analysis of the Data	
3:45 – 4:15 p.m.	Not in this training manual	Planning Other Steps: • Baseline Results Presentation to the NGOs, to Donors, and to Other Stakeholders • Qualitative Community Assessments • Health Facility Assessments	

Sample Agenda Module 6 (Monitoring and Evaluation Surveys): Tabulation and Data Analysis Workshop

Day 1

Time	Module and Session	Topic	Responsible
8:00 – 8:15 a.m.		Opening: Welcome Back	
8:15 – 8:30 a.m.		New Participant Introduction/Logistical Arrangements	
8:30 – 8:50 a.m.		Reviewing the Agenda for the Tabulation Workshop	
8:50 – 9:00 a.m.		Reviewing the Training Flow-Chart	
9:00 – 9:30 a.m.	M6/S1	Fieldwork Debriefing • Number of SAs in Which 19 Sets of Interviews Have Been Completed • Number of SAs with Data Collection Remaining—if Any • Confirmation that All Completed Sets of Questionnaires Have Been Brought to the Workshop • Contingency Plan for Finishing Tabulation of Remaining Questionnaires	

Day 1 (continued)

Time	Module and Session	Topic	Responsible
9:30 – 9:45 a.m.		• Tea/Coffee Break	
9:45 – 10:15 a.m.	M6/S1	• Lesson Learned During Data Collection: What Went Well and What Was Challenging	
10:15 – 11:15 a.m.	M6/S2	• Agreement on Correct Answers to the Questionnaires	
11:15 – 11:20 a.m.	M6/S2	Purpose of Tabulation	
11:20 – 12:00 p.m.	M6/S2	How to Use the Tabulation Tables: Reviewing the • SA Results Table • Variables Not Included in the Tabulation Tables (Filter Questions)	
12:00 – 1:00 p.m.		Lunch	
1:00 – 2:30 p.m.	M6/S2	Two Exercises: Using the Tabulation Tables to: • Enter Results for One Indicator in Each SA • Reviewing The Work of Each NGO • Repeating the Above Steps with a Second Indicator	
2:30 – 3:45 p.m.	M6/S2	**Tabulation Starts In Stages**	
3:45 – 4:00 p.m.		Tea/Coffee Break	
4:00 – 5:00 p.m.	M6/S2	Continue Tabulation in Stages	

Day 2

Time	Module and Session	Topic	Responsible
8:00 – 9:45 a.m.	M6/S2	Continue Tabulation in Stages	
9:45 – 10:00 a.m.		Tea/Coffee Break	
10:00 – 12:00 p.m.	M6/S2	Continue Tabulation in Stages	
12:00 – 1:00 p.m.		Lunch	
1:00 – 5:00 p.m.	M6/S2	Continue Tabulation in Stages	

Day 3

Time	Module and Session	Topic	Responsible
8:00 – 9:45 a.m.	M6/S2	Continue Tabulation in Stages	
9:45 – 10:00 a.m.		Tea/Coffee Break	
10:00 – 12:00 p.m.	M6/S2	Continue Tabulation in Stages	
12:00 – 1:00 p.m.		Lunch	
1:00 – 2:00 p.m.	M6/S3	How To Analyze LQAS Data and Identify Priorities Using the SA Results Tables and the Summary Tables: • Summary Table • How to Calculate Average Coverage and Why it is Important • Reviewing Coverage Targets Set for Key Indicators • Priorities Within an Individual SA When Considering Several Indicators Using Average Coverage and Performance Benchmarks • Priorities Among Several SAs When Considering One Indicator Using Average Coverage and Performance Benchmarks	
2:00 – 3:00 p.m.	M6/S3	Preparing a Monitoring and Evaluation Survey Report: • Purpose • Basic Outline: Data Analysis and Program. Planning Implications Setting Annual Goals	
3:00 – 3:15 p.m.		Tea/Coffee Break	
3:15 – 3:45 p.m.	Not in this training manual	Planning Next Steps: • Archiving Data in a Computer Data Based • Project-Wide Analysis of the Data	
3:45 – 4:15 p.m.	Not in this training manual	Planning Other Steps: • Monitoring and Evaluation Results Presentation to the NGOs, to Donors, and to Other Stakeholders • Qualitative Community Assessments • Health Facility Assessments	

Appendix 2: Dealing with More than One Respondent Type—Parallel Sampling

Identifying Interviewees

One of your most important challenges when carrying out a survey is deciding who you will interview. In community health projects the most typical groupings of people you could interview are in the following list.

Grouping	Type of Project
Women 15-49 Years of Age	• HIV/AIDS/STIs • Information women at-large in the community should know, like safe motherhood and other reproductive health information.
Women 15-49 Years of Age Not Pregnant	Family planning
Men 15-49 or 15-54 Years of Age	• HIV/AIDS/STIs • Information men at-large in the community should know, like safe motherhood and other reproductive health information. • Family planning
Mothers of Children 0-11 Months of Age	• Antenatal care, intra-partum, post-natal care. • Newborn care
Mothers of Children 12-23 Months of Age	• Vaccinations and Vitamin A (for the child) • Continuing breastfeeding
Either Mothers of Children 0-11 Months or Mothers of Children 12-23 Months of Age	• Knowledge of how to treat children with diarrhea or respiratory infection • Child Growth Monitoring • Nutrition
Sub-Grouping	**Type of Project**
Children of Mothers of Children 0-23 months sick in the last 2 weeks	Management of children sick with diarrhea or respiratory infections or fever
Mothers of Children 0-5 months	Exclusive Breastfeeding
Mothers of Children 6-9 months or 6-11 months	Complementary Breastfeeding

To choose a grouping of people to interview you have to decide who you expect the project to affect. By interviewing them, you can then determine whether your project is having a beneficial effect.

Interviewing Sub-Groups of Interviewees

When using LQAS methods it is ideal to ask each question in a survey to everyone in the age group who is interviewed. Some questions, however, you can only ask to a sub-group of interviewees. Try to minimize the number of questions that you ask to subgroups of interviewees.

For example, when you assess the vaccination program you ask to see the vaccination card of every child who is aged 12-23 months. Therefore, every mother is interviewed who has a child in this age range. When using LQAS you would interview 19 mothers in each SA with children in this age range. Then you would be able to compare each SA by the vaccination status of the children who live there. This approach is different than some other approaches that sample children 0-23 months but then assess only a part of the sample, namely, children 12-23 months.

However, if a project is training mothers to give their children oral rehydration therapy, some questions in the survey would be asked only of mothers whose children had diarrhea in the last 2 weeks. Since not every child has been sick in the last 2 weeks, these questions would be asked to a sub-group of mothers rather than mothers of all children.

The data collected in sub-groups has less statistical power than the data collected from all of the interviewees. As a result it is best to minimize the number of questions asked of a sub-group of interviewees. With questions asked of sub-groups, you often cannot compare performance of the SAs since there is not enough information in each SA to make an LQAS judgment. In this situation, it is better to calculate average coverage for the entire project catchment area, and not to use LQAS decision rules to compare the different SAs.

Parallel Sampling and Developing a Questionnaire

Frequently, you will need to interview more than one grouping of interviewees. In many child survival projects we interview at least 2 groupings:

- Mothers of children 0-11 months of age
- Mothers of children 12-23 months of age.

It is better to interview 2 samples rather than to interview 1 sample of mothers of children 0–23 months. The main reason is that the sub-groupings would be too small to produce accurate results. For example, in a single sample you would have at most 25% of the interviewees to assess exclusive breastfeeding, and only half of the sample to assess vaccination coverage—two very important activities. This is because only the 0-5 age group (a quarter of the 0–23 month age group) is assessed for exclusive breastfeeding. And only children 12–23 months (50% of the 0-23 month age group) is assessed for their vaccination status.

Questions that are related to the condition of the child rather than to his/her age should be put in all of the questionnaires. For example, it is a great advantage to include the questions about treatment of sick children in the questionnaires asked of both the mothers of children 0-11 months and mothers of children 12-23 months. The reason is that you can add together the information obtained from both questionnaires and have data that is statistically more powerful and more meaningful.

Remember –the type of respondent depends on the health intervention. Identify your respondents as soon as possible when you plan a survey.

How to Parallel Sample
Let's assume that your community health program intends to
- increase the percentage of pregnant women who attend at least one antenatal care visit,
- improve newborn care,
- increase vaccination coverage,
- improve mothers' skills in preparing oral rehydration solution,
- improve the treatment of children with diarrhea, and
- increase the percentage of women who use a family planning method.

Using the table above you would prepare three short questionnaires to interview three groups in the community, namely, mothers of children 0-11 months, mothers of children 12-23 months, and women 15-49 years of age who are not pregnant.

To parallel sample, follow these steps:
1. Go to each community where you have to take one of the 19 LQAS samples. You learned how to do this already using a sampling frame.
2. Randomly select one household in the community, as you were taught, and go to it.
3. If a woman 15-49 years lives there then use the woman's questionnaire in that household.

4. If there is either a mother of a child 0-11 months or 12-23 months then use that questionnaire in that household too. If there is no mother with a child in this age group then go to the next house.

Continue going to the closest house until all three questionnaires have been used. You cannot sample a mother of a child 0-11 months and mother of child 12-23 months in the same household. The reason is that because you are assessing mothers' treatment of their sick children you have be sure that all of your mothers live in different households. Mothers who live in the same household may treat their child in the same way. Therefore it is better to always sample mothers of children who live in different households.

Appendix 3: Decision rules for an LQAS sample of 19. Upper thresholds are average coverage/coverage targets range from 20-95%. Lower thresholds range from 0-75%. Corresponding producer and consumer risks (alpha and beta errors) are included. Optimal decision rules are highlighted.

Lower Threshold	20%	25%	30%	35%	40%	45%	50%	55%	60%	65%	70%	75%	80%	85%	90%	95%
0%	1 / 0.014 / 0.000	2 / 0.031 / 0.000	3 / 0.046 / 0.000	3 / 0.017 / 0.000												
5%		3 / 0.111 / 0.067	3 / 0.046 / 0.067	4 / 0.059 / 0.013	4 / 0.023 / 0.013											
10%				4 / 0.059 / 0.067	5 / 0.070 / 0.035	5 / 0.028 / 0.035	6 / 0.032 / 0.009									
15%					5 / 0.070 / 0.144	6 / 0.078 / 0.054	6 / 0.032 / 0.054	7 / 0.034 / 0.016								
20%						7 / 0.173 / 0.068	7 / 0.084 / 0.068	7 / 0.034 / 0.068	8 / 0.035 / 0.023							
25%							8 / 0.180 / 0.077	8 / 0.087 / 0.077	8 / 0.035 / 0.077	9 / 0.035 / 0.029						
30%							8 / 0.180 / 0.182	9 / 0.184 / 0.084	9 / 0.088 / 0.084	9 / 0.035 / 0.084	10 / 0.033 / 0.033					
35%								9 / 0.184 / 0.185	10 / 0.186 / 0.087	10 / 0.087 / 0.087	10 / 0.033 / 0.087	11 / 0.029 / 0.035				
40%									10 / 0.186 / 0.185	11 / 0.185 / 0.088	11 / 0.084 / 0.088	12 / 0.077 / 0.035	12 / 0.023 / 0.035			
45%										11 / 0.185 / 0.186	11 / 0.084 / 0.184	12 / 0.077 / 0.087	13 / 0.068 / 0.034	13 / 0.016 / 0.034		
50%											12 / 0.182 / 0.180	12 / 0.077 / 0.180	13 / 0.068 / 0.084	14 / 0.054 / 0.032	14 / 0.009 / 0.032	
55%												13 / 0.175 / 0.173	14 / 0.163 / 0.078	14 / 0.054 / 0.078	15 / 0.035 / 0.028	16 / 0.013 / 0.008
60%													14 / 0.163 / 0.163	15 / 0.144 / 0.070	15 / 0.035 / 0.070	16 / 0.013 / 0.023
65%														15 / 0.144 / 0.150	16 / 0.115 / 0.059	16 / 0.013 / 0.059
70%															16 / 0.115 / 0.133	17 / 0.067 / 0.046
75%																17 / 0.067 / 0.111

AVERAGE COVERAGE (Baselines, Monitoring and Evaluation) / ANNUAL COVERAGE TARGET (Monitoring and Evaluation)

What Is an Alpha and Beta Error?

Alpha and beta errors tell you how often your judgments will be wrong about whether an SA has reached a performance benchmark. The LQAS Table, you have been taught to use, has performance benchmarks as the top row. The benchmarks range from 20% to 95%.

Let's assume that you are using an LQAS sample size of 19. Let's also assume that your performance benchmark is 80% measles vaccination coverage. As you will remember, the LQAS decision rule is 13 (Now would be a good time to refer to your table to verify that the decision rule is 13!). Let's assume that you are assessing SA-#1 and that according to a census we already know that measles vaccination coverage is exactly 80%.

In this example, the alpha error is less than 10% for a sample of 19, a decision rule of 13 and a benchmark of 80%. This is noted in the footnote of the LQAS table. The exact alpha error is noted in the table presented above, namely, 0.068. This means that by using the LQAS decision rule of 13, when you assess an SA that truly has 80% coverage, more than 90 times out of 100 you will correctly judge that it has reached the benchmark. In other words, more than 90 times out of 100 in a sample of 19, 13 or more of the children will have a measles vaccination. In only 6.8 times out of 100 will less than 13 of the children be vaccinated – this is the alpha error.

Beta errors judge whether the sample is identifying areas that are far below 80%. When we constructed the LQAS table, we assumed that supervisors had to be very certain they would identify an SA that is 30 percentage points below the performance benchmark. So if the benchmark is 80%, LQAS will be very sensitive to an SA that has 50% coverage (80%-50%=30%). In LQAS we refer to this as the lower threshold.

Using the LQAS table, the beta error is less than 10% for a sample of 19, a decision rule of 13 and a performance benchmark of 80%. The exact beta error is noted in the table presented above, namely, 0.084. This means that by using the LQAS decision rule of 13, when you assess an SA that truly has 50% coverage, more than 90 times out of 100 you will correctly judge that it has NOT reached the benchmark. In other words, more than 90 times out of 100 in a sample of 19, less than 13 children will have a measles vaccination. Only 8.4 times out of 100 will more than 13 of the children be vaccinated – this is the beta error.

If the lower threshold, used for setting the beta error, was located 20 percentage points from the performance benchmark, instead of 30 percentage points, then the beta error would be higher. If you look at the table above for performance benchmark of 80% and a lower threshold of 60% you will notice that the error is 0.163. This is twice as high as 0.084 although it is still low.

Why Use a Sample of 19?

Now that you know about alpha and beta errors we can answer the question of why we recommend that you most often use a sample of 19 rather than a larger sample.

Any sample that is less than 19 will have alpha or beta errors that are greater than 10%. By keeping error less than 10% we are consistent with a statistical convention, namely, to try to keep error to less than 10%.

Similarly, by increasing the sample size you create more work and do not necessarily reduce the number of SAs that you incorrectly assess. Here is an example. Let's assume that we have 32 SAs and that exactly 16 have 80% coverage and 16 have 50% coverage. Also, let's assume that we are using two LQAS sample to judge whether they have reached the performance benchmark of 80% measles vaccination coverage. As the table below shows, the same number of SAs will be incorrectly misclassified regardless of whether the same is 19 or half again as large.

Sample of 28	
16 adequate SAs (80% coverage) X .039 alpha error 0.624 or 1 misclassified as poor	16 sub-standard SAs (50% coverage) X .044 beta error 0.704 or 1 misclassified as adequate
Sample of 19	
16 adequate SAs (80% coverage) X .068 error 1.08 or 1 misclassified as poor	16 sub-standard SAs (50% coverage) X .084 beta error 1.344 or 1 misclassified as adequate

Appendix 4: Additional Random Number Table 1

87172 43062 39719 10020 32722 86545 86985 04962 54546 23138 62135 55870 97083 67875
28900 50851 30543 89185 16747 95104 49852 26467 58869 79053 06894 23975 34902 23587
86248 71156 55044 13045 33161 95604 57876 23367 10768 78193 60477 70307 06498 48793
10531 51391 41884 69759 32741 70072 01902 96656 90584 59263 49995 27235 40055 20917
02481 90230 81978 39127 93335 74259 25856 52838 49847 69042 85964 78159 40374 49658
23988 13019 78830 17069 58267 69796 94329 34050 25622 55349 10403 93790 77631 74261
37137 47689 82466 24243 10756 54009 44053 74870 28352 66389 38729 80349 50509 56465
38230 82039 34158 90149 82948 60686 27962 39306 53826 47852 76144 38812 76939 03119
98745 08288 19108 84791 58470 59415 45456 44839 86274 25091 42809 56707 47169 95273
44653 58412 91751 14954 87949 81399 51105 29718 82780 11262 23712 99782 42829 26308
88386 66621 16648 19217 52375 05417 26136 05952 71958 25744 52021 20225 01377 47012
50660 58138 01695 69351 25445 20797 74079 60851 47634 36633 93999 96345 58484 12506
36732 74234 84240 46924 62744 39238 78397 60869 26426 55588 56963 59506 17293 45096
34187 78277 83678 34754 46616 45250 25291 04999 19717 60324 66915 03473 98329 82447
26095 98131 79362 39530 53870 87445 26277 90551 28604 39865 40686 05435 74511 69866
00067 74289 20706 74076 28206 36960 09231 82988 57062 35331 08212 68111 52199 05065
42104 26434 30953 15259 76676 63339 75664 23993 63538 34968 47655 44553 61982 13296
82580 46580 87292 23226 21865 60338 04115 33807 38395 98484 40387 69877 24910 13317
89266 14764 17681 68663 66030 12931 17372 35601 63805 55739 42705 30549 31697 33478
47100 92329 89435 69974 40783 52649 93444 41317 02749 19052 34647 92814 88046 34020
59566 26527 44706 85670 96223 36275 82013 82673 60955 62617 90214 24589 59715 57612
10946 24676 66513 56743 96911 89042 08263 70753 89045 39189 04306 06090 94515 17772
34013 69250 27977 84597 55192 65088 55739 35953 18533 39339 78037 32827 68269 69218
21606 11751 30073 71431 53569 27865 90215 34772 21779 11734 64313 49764 30816 56852
56620 92612 77157 90231 90144 29781 01683 52503 60080 73703 70080 80686 47379 33279
49238 90475 84356 87159 21222 40106 02671 52684 38514 68434 16407 58164 13341 48142
50738 21999 73539 51802 78179 27872 57937 29696 67783 29373 96563 74619 77099 17190
58761 21571 71692 19723 25088 10483 71430 47068 78378 80237 32113 09381 62931 29243
55335 71937 22025 33538 04648 74232 57839 62431 61835 04784 06732 34202 93497 72070
26515 31143 83795 78445 32869 31489 81587 90354 97672 70106 35008 37899 36246 97805
32625 36806 00082 26902 26250 28919 38054 49027 22209 42696 46980 17065 61288 30208
20311 96089 20141 30362 04980 32703 04202 91080 28660 89691 84660 73433 70169 11273
10941 73003 87930 85620 06956 38719 88711 61454 64076 13316 02203 54437 54306 78229
56982 46636 34070 30803 39095 80387 08971 25067 07377 70704 13629 68474 99229 05535
14661 10670 15811 00454 81124 46977 89983 48836 48182 17054 06344 24267 16686 21401
52760 78118 23277 29760 00099 97325 54762 43117 73199 19621 24599 11030 64809 35088
48874 20831 02286 73635 93771 54264 49801 22653 01524 84621 91023 64028 29278 15987
44817 77408 48447 25934 22912 43086 68126 92970 91833 26418 72454 97636 94593 07880
17896 79375 70883 70135 21589 51181 71969 32951 35036 17219 27357 96517 55307 84470
27166 22347 92146 92189 16301 15747 72837 59174 75024 39459 54910 95335 95013 47068
13665 30490 63583 73098 19976 03001 94645 40476 43617 85698 66512 42759 20973 98759
58644 73840 08103 97926 57340 63077 08114 10031 35668 21740 33787 44756 20527 65367
72570 36278 06602 56406 85679 85529 08576 50874 59706 01019 29980 56742 05356 04810
92041 68829 02163 59918 83041 71241 90678 79835 86324 13075 29913 99831 25688 53648
71240 74119 53090 23693 14007 90107 68804 54927 68964 26535 28184 21630 12362 67990

Additional Random Number Table 2

```
87172 43062 39719 10020 32722 86545 86985 04962 54546 23138 62135 55870 97083 67875
28900 50851 30543 89185 16747 95104 49852 26467 58869 79053 06894 23975 34902 23587
86248 71156 55044 13045 33161 95604 57876 23367 10768 78193 60477 70307 06498 48793
10531 51391 41884 69759 32741 70072 01902 96656 90584 59263 49995 27235 40055 20917
02481 90230 81978 39127 93335 74259 25856 52838 49847 69042 85964 78159 40374 49658
23988 13019 78830 17069 58267 69796 94329 34050 25622 55349 10403 93790 77631 74261
37137 47689 82466 24243 10756 54009 44053 74870 28352 66389 38729 80349 50509 56465
38230 82039 34158 90149 82948 60686 27962 39306 53826 47852 76144 38812 76939 03119
98745 08288 19108 84791 58470 59415 45456 44839 86274 25091 42809 56707 47169 95273
44653 58412 91751 14954 87949 81399 51105 29718 82780 11262 23712 99782 42829 26308
88386 66621 16648 19217 52375 05417 26136 05952 71958 25744 52021 20225 01377 47012
50660 58138 01695 69351 25445 20797 74079 60851 47634 36633 93999 96345 58484 12506
36732 74234 84240 46924 62744 39238 78397 60869 26426 55588 56963 59506 17293 45096
34187 78277 83678 34754 46616 45250 25291 04999 19717 60324 66915 03473 98329 82447
26095 98131 79362 39530 53870 87445 26277 90551 28604 39865 40686 05435 74511 69866
00067 74289 20706 74076 28206 36960 09231 82988 57062 35331 08212 68111 52199 05065
42104 26434 30953 15259 76676 63339 75664 23993 63538 34968 47655 44553 61982 13296
82580 46580 87292 23226 21865 60338 04115 33807 38395 98484 40387 69877 24910 13317
89266 14764 17681 68663 66030 12931 17372 35601 63805 55739 42705 30549 31697 33478
47100 92329 89435 69974 40783 52649 93444 41317 02749 19052 34647 92814 88046 34020
59566 26527 44706 85670 96223 36275 82013 82673 60955 62617 90214 24589 59715 57612
10946 24676 66513 56743 96911 89042 08263 70753 89045 39189 04306 06090 94515 17772
34013 69250 27977 84597 55192 65088 55739 35953 18533 39339 78037 32827 68269 69218
21606 11751 30073 71431 53569 27865 90215 34772 21779 11734 64313 49764 30816 56852
56620 92612 77157 90231 90144 29781 01683 52503 60080 73703 70080 80686 47379 33279
49238 90475 84356 87159 21222 40106 02671 52684 38514 68434 16407 58164 13341 48142
50738 21999 73539 51802 78179 27872 57937 29696 67783 29373 96563 74619 77099 17190
58761 21571 71692 19723 25088 10483 71430 47068 78378 80237 32113 09381 62931 29243
55335 71937 22025 33538 04648 74232 57839 62431 61835 04784 06732 34202 93497 72070
26515 31143 83795 78445 32869 31489 81587 90354 97672 70106 35008 37899 36246 97805
32625 36806 00082 26902 26250 28919 38054 49027 22209 42696 46980 17065 61288 30208
20311 96089 20141 30362 04980 32703 04202 91080 28660 89691 84660 73433 70169 11273
10941 73003 87930 85620 06956 38719 88711 61454 64076 13316 02203 54437 54306 78229
56982 46636 34070 30803 39095 80387 08971 25067 07377 70704 13629 68474 99229 05535
14661 10670 15811 00454 81124 46977 89983 48836 48182 17054 06344 24267 16686 21401
52760 78118 23277 29760 00099 97325 54762 43117 73199 19621 24599 11030 64809 35088
48874 20831 02286 73635 93771 54264 49801 22653 01524 84621 91023 64028 29278 15987
44817 77408 48447 25934 22912 43086 68126 92970 91833 26418 72454 97636 94593 07880
17896 79375 70883 70135 21589 51181 71969 32951 35036 17219 27357 96517 55307 84470
27166 22347 92146 92189 16301 15747 72837 59174 75024 39459 54910 95335 95013 47068
13665 30490 63583 73098 19976 03001 94645 40476 43617 85698 66512 42759 20973 98759
58644 73840 08103 97926 57340 63077 08114 10031 35668 21740 33787 44756 20527 65367
72570 36278 06602 56406 85679 85529 08576 50874 59706 01019 29980 56742 05356 04810
92041 68829 02163 59918 83041 71241 90678 79835 86324 13075 29913 99831 25688 53648
71240 74119 53090 23693 14007 90107 68804 54927 68964 26535 28184 21630 12362 67990
```

Additional Random Number Table 3

```
87172 43062 39719 10020 32722 86545 86985 04962 54546 23138 62135 55870 97083 67875
28900 50851 30543 89185 16747 95104 49852 26467 58869 79053 06894 23975 34902 23587
86248 71156 55044 13045 33161 95604 57876 23367 10768 78193 60477 70307 06498 48793
10531 51391 41884 69759 32741 70072 01902 96656 90584 59263 49995 27235 40055 20917
02481 90230 81978 39127 93335 74259 25856 52838 49847 69042 85964 78159 40374 49658
23988 13019 78830 17069 58267 69796 94329 34050 25622 55349 10403 93790 77631 74261
37137 47689 82466 24243 10756 54009 44053 74870 28352 66389 38729 80349 50509 56465
38230 82039 34158 90149 82948 60686 27962 39306 53826 47852 76144 38812 76939 03119
98745 08288 19108 84791 58470 59415 45456 44839 86274 25091 42809 56707 47169 95273
44653 58412 91751 14954 87949 81399 51105 29718 82780 11262 23712 99782 42829 26308
88386 66621 16648 19217 52375 05417 26136 05952 71958 25744 52021 20225 01377 47012
50660 58138 01695 69351 25445 20797 74079 60851 47634 36633 93999 96345 58484 12506
36732 74234 84240 46924 62744 39238 78397 60869 26426 55588 56963 59506 17293 45096
34187 78277 83678 34754 46616 45250 25291 04999 19717 60324 66915 03473 98329 82447
26095 98131 79362 39530 53870 87445 26277 90551 28604 39865 40686 05435 74511 69866
00067 74289 20706 74076 28206 36960 09231 82988 57062 35331 08212 68111 52199 05065
42104 26434 30953 15259 76676 63339 75664 23993 63538 34968 47655 44553 61982 13296
82580 46580 87292 23226 21865 60338 04115 33807 38395 98484 40387 69877 24910 13317
89266 14764 17681 68663 66030 12931 17372 35601 63805 55739 42705 30549 31697 33478
47100 92329 89435 69974 40783 52649 93444 41317 02749 19052 34647 92814 88046 34020
59566 26527 44706 85670 96223 36275 82013 82673 60955 62617 90214 24589 59715 57612
10946 24676 66513 56743 96911 89042 08263 70753 89045 39189 04306 06090 94515 17772
34013 69250 27977 84597 55192 65088 55739 35953 18533 39339 78037 32827 68269 69218
21606 11751 30073 71431 53569 27865 90215 34772 21779 11734 64313 49764 30816 56852
56620 92612 77157 90231 90144 29781 01683 52503 60080 73703 70080 80686 47379 33279
49238 90475 84356 87159 21222 40106 02671 52684 38514 68434 16407 58164 13341 48142
50738 21999 73539 51802 78179 27872 57937 29696 67783 29373 96563 74619 77099 17190
58761 21571 71692 19723 25088 10483 71430 47068 78378 80237 32113 09381 62931 29243
55335 71937 22025 33538 04648 74232 57839 62431 61835 04784 06732 34202 93497 72070
26515 31143 83795 78445 32869 31489 81587 90354 97672 70106 35008 37899 36246 97805
32625 36806 00082 26902 26250 28919 38054 49027 22209 42696 46980 17065 61288 30208
20311 96089 20141 30362 04980 32703 04202 91080 28660 89691 84660 73433 70169 11273
10941 73003 87930 85620 06956 38719 88711 61454 64076 13316 02203 54437 54306 78229
56982 46636 34070 30803 39095 80387 08971 25067 07377 70704 13629 68474 99229 05535
14661 10670 15811 00454 81124 46977 89983 48836 48182 17054 06344 24267 16686 21401
52760 78118 23277 29760 00099 97325 54762 43117 73199 19621 24599 11030 64809 35088
48874 20831 02286 73635 93771 54264 49801 22653 01524 84621 91023 64028 29278 15987
44817 77408 48447 25934 22912 43086 68126 92970 91833 26418 72454 97636 94593 07880
17896 79375 70883 70135 21589 51181 71969 32951 35036 17219 27357 96517 55307 84470
27166 22347 92146 92189 16301 15747 72837 59174 75024 39459 54910 95335 95013 47068
13665 30490 63583 73098 19976 03001 94645 40476 43617 85698 66512 42759 20973 98759
58644 73840 08103 97926 57340 63077 08114 10031 35668 21740 33787 44756 20527 65367
72570 36278 06602 56406 85679 85529 08576 50874 59706 01019 29980 56742 05356 04810
92041 68829 02163 59918 83041 71241 90678 79835 86324 13075 29913 99831 25688 53648
71240 74119 53090 23693 14007 90107 68804 54927 68964 26535 28184 21630 12362 67990
```

Appendix 5: Additional Community Scenarios

Selecting the first house in urban blocks or districts

- Block #54 was selected as the approximate location for the first interview.
- The interviewer arrives, and now what? How do you select a house for the first interview?
- HINT: Number the houses and choose one randomly. Or you could choose one of the four sides randomly and then number the houses on that side only. Then choose one of them randomly.

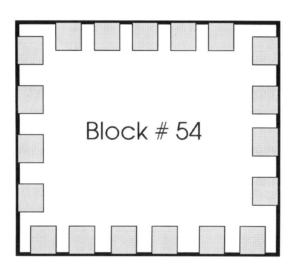

Selecting the first house: <u>crowded</u> blocks or districts

- Block #9 was selected as the approximate location for the first interview.
- The interviewer arrives, and now what?
- HINT: Divide the Block into four quadrants or sectors. Choose one sector randomly. Count the number of houses in that sector and select one house randomly.

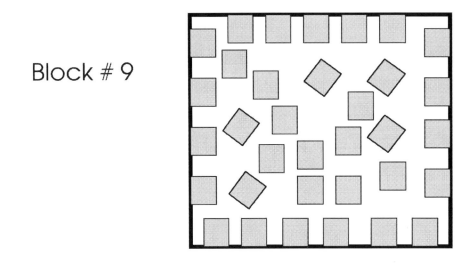

Block # 9

Selecting the first house: An apartment building

- Building #73 was selected as the approximate location for the first interview.

- It is an apartment building.

- The interviewer arrives, and now what?

- HINT: Number the floors of the apartment building.

    - Choose one floor randomly.

    - Count the number of doors on that floor. Choose one door randomly.

    - If you cannot use the rule of "go to the closest door" since all doors are next to each other or equally close, then choose one rule before beginning your search, such as, "Always go to the right."

    - Similarly, if you find no one on the floor you can interview, choose one rule before beginning your search instructing you to go up one floor or down one floor.

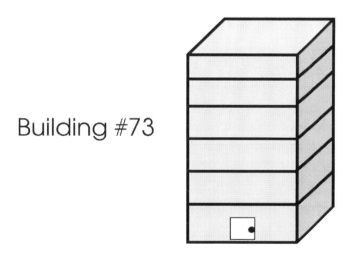

Building #73

Selecting the first house: Apartments and houses together

- Block #27 was selected as the approximate location for the first interview.
- There are both apartments and houses in this block.
- The interviewer arrives, and now what?
- HINT: In complex situations like this one, the simplest solution may be to count all of the houses/doors in the selected block and choose one randomly. You could estimate the number of doors in an apartment building by counting the number of doors on one floor and then multiplying this number by the number of floors in the building.

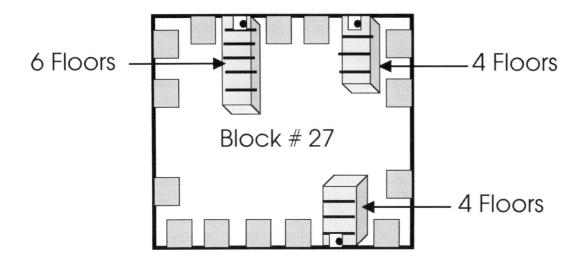

Appendix 6: How to Calculate Weighted Coverage and Confidence Intervals

Calculating a weighted average is more precise than an unweighted, crude measure. This calculation takes into account that not all SAs are of the same size. The contribution each SA makes to the calculation of the average should be related to its size. Although a weighted average is more accurate than a crude measure, in most cases it is only slightly more precise. Therefore, if you are able only to present a crude average, simply do so and note this decision in your reports.

Data can be weighted by SA population sizes using the *direct adjustment method*. While weighting is not needed when making LQAS judgements of an SA, it can be used when aggregating the data to calculate coverage for an entire catchment area or geographical area. Let's assume that a sample of 19 interview sets were carried out in each SA regardless of the SA population size and the number of SAs in the catchment area. Without weighting, a sample of 19 can potentially either overestimate or underestimate the coverage estimate. Weighting the data allows us to remove this distortion.

Calculating Weighted Coverage Proportions with a Confidence Interval by Hand

Most Ministries of Health at national and regional levels, and District Health Management Teams, calculate estimates of coverage for various interventions.

While LQAS data are quite useful for identifying SAs and interventions that are reaching coverage targets and those which are not, these same data can be used to calculate coverage proportions. This, however, is not the primary purpose for collecting LQAS data. Nevertheless, they can be used in this way. And it is a useful bi-product since the Ministry of Health and donors often want this information. When LQAS data are added together to calculate a coverage proportion, they are treated as a stratified random sample.

To calculate coverage with LQAS, use the example presented in Table 1.

Table 1: Adding together 5 LQAS SAs to Calculate an Overall Coverage Estimate							
Health Center (SA)	SA Sample Size = n	Number Correct=C	$p = C/n$ =mini%	N	$wt = N_i / \Sigma N$	$wt * p$ or $wt *$ mini%
Thika	19	7	0.37	10,718	0.245	0.09
Kiambu	19	14	0.74	6,379	0.146	0.108
Muthari	19	5	0.26	9,379	0.215	0.056
Nyeri	19	16	0.84	9,731	0.223	0.187
Naivasha	19	4	0.21	7,500	0.172	0.036
Totals	95			43,707		
					Coverage =	0.478

Let's assume you are assessing a Growth Monitoring and Promotion program. Column 1 lists 5 Health Centers (SAs) in a project catchment area. Column 2 is the sample size of each SA (19 in this case). Column 3 is the number of women in the sample that had up-to-date growth charts. Column 4 is a mini-coverage proportion (p) for each SA. This is calculated by using the number of women in the sample with up-to-date growth charts as a numerator, and the number of women in the sample as the denominator (which is 19). Therefore, 7/19 = 0.37 in the case of Thika. Column 5 is the size of the population in each SA; this can be an estimate because wide fluctuations in this number have little influence on the overall calculation. Column 6 is a weight which is calculated as the population in each SA divided by the total population of all the SAs in the entire catchment area. Therefore, the weight for Thika is 10,718/43,707 = 0.245. Column 7 is the final calculation, which multiplies the *weight* and the mini-coverage proportion in each SA. Adding these numbers together gives the overall coverage estimate for the catchment area. In this case, the coverage in the catchment area is 47.8%.

The final step in measuring a coverage proportion is to calculate the confidence interval (CI). This measure is needed because the coverage calculation is an estimate and will not be precise. A 95% CI is the range in which we are 95% confident that the true coverage is within. Table 2 demonstrates this calculation.

Table 2: Calculating a Confidence Interval for a Coverage Proportion for a District Having 5 SAs

Health Centers (SA)	wt^2	$p \times q$	$\dfrac{wt^2 \times (pq)}{n}$
Thika	0.060	0.233	0.001
Kiambu	0.021	0.194	0.000
Muthari	0.046	0.194	0.000
Nyeri	0.050	0.133	0.000
Naivasha	0.029	0.166	0.000
Totals			0.002

CI = (1.96 x SQRT(0.002)) = ± 0.083

Column 2 uses the weight from Table 1 and then squares it. Column 3 uses the value *p*, the mini-coverage proportion referred to in the previous table. The value of *q* is (1 – p). The last column multiplies the values of columns 2 and 3, and divides them by 19 (the sample size, n). This procedure results in very small values that have more than 3 decimal places. That is why some row values are 0.000. The actual values of these very small decimals are located in the fourth decimal place, which you cannot see. When they are added together they result in a value of 0.002. The final step is to multiply the square root of 0.002 by 1.96; the resulting value, ±8.3%, is the confidence interval.

Therefore, the coverage in the project catchment area is 47.8%, ±8.3%. In other words, we are 95% confident that the true coverage in this district is between 39.5% and 56.1%.

Calculating Weighted Coverage and Confidence Intervals with a Computer

The simplest way to calculate a weighted coverage and confidence interval is using CSAMPLE in the EPIINFO program. This is statistical software that is widely distributed without cost by the Centers for Disease Control. If you want a copy, go to http:///www.CDC.gov to search for either the DOS or WINDOWS version. This section presumes you are using the DOS version.

On the first screen in EPIINFO, locate the 10th option under *Programs*. You will see CSAMPLE. Once you load your data set, you come to a complex screen with several highlighted boxes. You need to consider only 3 of them: MAIN, STRATA, and WEIGHT.

MAIN = the variable or indicator you are analyzing

STRATA = the variable name that has the code for each SA. Each SA should have its own code number. If there are 5 SAs then the numbers should range from 1 to 5.

WEIGHT = the weight for each SA. The easiest way to add this information is after your data have been entered and cleaned. Then, prior to analysis, write a program that looks like this:

```
Read [filename].rec
Define weight #####
Let WEIGHT = 0
If SA=1 then  WEIGHT = 10718
If SA=2 then  WEIGHT = 6379
If SA=3 then  WEIGHT = 9379
If SA=4 then  WEIGHT = 9731
If SA=5 then  WEIGHT = 7500
Route [new filename].rec
Write recfile
```

Once you run this little program your dataset will have a permanent new variable called WEIGHT in a new file that you can use for analyzing in CSAMPLE.

How Many SAs Should I Have?

A frequently asked question during a program planning is: How many SAs should I design into the program? Throughout the Training Guide, we have recommended at least 5 SAs. The reason is that with 5 SAs you will always have a coverage proportion calculated with a total sample of 95 (19 x 5 = 95). This sample size will have a confidence interval that will always be less than ±10%.

If you have less than 5 SAs the confidence interval increases. If you have more than 5 SAs, the confidence interval decreases. This means that coverage estimates with less than 5 SAs are less precise. Similarly, coverage estimates with more than 5 SAs are increasingly more precise. The following table presents several scenarios with different numbers of SAs so you can see how the confidence intervals change. The tables try to maintain a coverage proportion of about 50% since the confidence interval is always widest when the coverage is 50%. These tables can help inform you about what the precision of coverage proportions will be depending on the number of SAs you have.

Although we recommend that you create at least 5 SAs, in practice, we have often used 4 SAs. The reason is that at that time in the lives of those projects, the manager thought that from a management point of view it made sense to divide their area into 4 SAs. It is important to be very practical when defining SAs. Each one should conform to a real management unit. This is important since the LQAS data will aid the manager of each SA to learn how well s/he is performing in comparison to other SAs.

Example 1: 8 Supervision Areas

SA	N	Corrects	mini %	N	wt	wt*(mini%)
1	19	7	0.368	10,718	0.16	0.06
2	19	14	0.737	6,379	0.09	0.07
3	19	5	0.263	9,379	0.14	0.04
4	19	16	0.842	9,731	0.14	0.12
5	19	6	0.316	7,500	0.11	0.04
6	19	9	0.474	8,000	0.12	0.06
7	19	10	0.526	7,500	0.11	0.06
8	19	10	0.526	8,000	0.12	0.06
	152	77		67,207	Weighted Coverage	0.500
					Confidence Interval =	0.073

Example 2: 6 Supervision Areas

Cohort	N	Corrects	mini %	N	wt	wt*(mini%)
1	19	7	0.368	10,718	0.21	0.08
2	19	14	0.737	6,379	0.12	0.09
3	19	5	0.263	9,379	0.18	0.05
4	19	16	0.842	9,731	0.19	0.16
5	19	6	0.316	7,500	0.15	0.05
6	19	10	0.526	8,000	0.15	0.08
	114	58		51,707	**Weighted Coverage**	**0.501**
					Confidence Interval =	**0.082**

Example 3: 5 Supervision Areas

Cohort	N	Corrects	mini %	N	wt	wt*(mini%)
1	19	7	0.368	10,718	0.25	0.09
2	19	14	0.737	6,379	0.15	0.11
3	19	5	0.263	9,379	0.21	0.06
4	19	16	0.842	9,731	0.22	0.19
5	19	6	0.316	7,500	0.17	0.05
	95	48		43,707	**Weighted Coverage**	**0.50**
					Confidence Interval =	**0.090**

Example 4: 4 Supervision Areas

Cohort	N	Corrects	mini %	N	wt	wt*(mini%)
1	19	7	0.368	10,718	0.30	0.11
2	19	14	0.737	6,379	0.18	0.13
3	19	6	0.316	9,379	0.26	0.08
4	19	13	0.684	9,731	0.27	0.18
	76	40		36,207	**Weighted Coverage**	**0.50**
					Confidence Interval =	**0.107**

Example 5: 3 Supervision Areas

Cohort	N	Corrects	mini %	N	wt	wt*(mini%)
1	19	9	0.474	10,718	0.40	0.19
2	19	14	0.737	6,379	0.24	0.18
3	19	7	0.368	9,379	0.35	0.13
	57	30		26,476	**Weighted Coverage**	**0.50**
					Confidence Interval =	**0.128**

Appendix 7: Example Tabulation Tables for Sub-Samples in which You Use Aggregate Measures Only

This section shows you 2 tabulation tables and 2 summary tables. One is for exclusive breastfeeding and the other concerns treatment of children who have had diarrhea in the last 2 weeks. We show you examples for these 2 activities because very many child survival programs include them as important components of their programs.

Both activities share one thing in common—rather than using all 19 samples, they only use part of them for analysis. These parts are called sub-groups. When exclusive breastfeeding is analyzed, you use the information collected from mothers of children 0–5 months of age. This means you would use about half of the children interviewed with the questionnaire intended for mothers of children 0–11 months of age.

The number of children who have had diarrhea in the last 2 weeks is entirely dependent on the prevalence of diarrhea. If diarrhea prevalence is 25%, then only a quarter of children 0–11 months and 12–23 months would be included in this assessment. It is for this reason that it is best to always include questions about sick children in both of these questionnaires.

Often when only a small part of a sample is used rather than the entire sample, you cannot use the LQAS table to analyze the data in a supervision area. The reason is that there is too little information.

In this situation the best thing to do is to analyze the information for the catchment area as a whole. To do this you add the information together to measure average coverage of exclusive breastfeeding, average diarrhea prevalence, and other averages related to the correct treatment of children who have had diarrhea in the last 2 weeks.

RESULTS TABLE FOR A MUNICIPALITY: Kwa-Zulu Natal, South Africa February 2002

Exclusive Breastfeeding --- Mothers of Children 0-11 Months

Municipality (Supervision Area): _____ Supervisor: _____

Number of the Supervision Area: _____

CORRECT=1
INCORRECT=0
SKIPPED=S
MISSING=X

NO.	INDICATOR	Code for the Correct Response (Review all responses of OTHER and include if appropriate)	1	2	3	4	5	6	7	8	9	10	11	12	13	14	15	16	17	18	19	Total N0. Correct (Excludes X & S)
SECTION 2: EXCLUSIVE BREASTFEEDING																						
	If the Child is 0–5 months mark a "1". ---- If child is 6–11 months mark an "S".																						
	Next Questions for Children 0–5 months ONLY -- Code next questions only if the above Row is coded as "1"																						
2A	Are you breastfeeding now?	YES																					
6A-M	Have you given [NAME] any of the foods or liquids in 6A-M in the last 24 hours? (If child is 6–11 months mark as "S")	NO must be recorded for all questions 6A through 6M																					
	Exclusive Breastfeeding (Mark an "S" if child is 6–11 months)	Both of the two above rows are correct																					

Appendix 7: Example Tabulation Tables for Sub-Samples

RESULTS TABLE FOR A MUNICIPALITY: Kwa-Zulu Natal, South Africa February 2002

Treatment of the Sick Child --- Mothers of Children 0-23 Months

CORRECT=1
INCORRECT=0
SKIPPED=S
MISSING=X

Municipality: _____ Supervisor: _____

NAME OR NUMBER OF THE SUPERVISION AREA: _____

Table Quest. No.	Quest. NO.	INDICATOR	Code for the Correct Response (Review all responses of OTHER and include if appropriate)	1	2	3	4	5	6	7	8	9	10	11	12	13	14	15	16	17	18	19	Total N0. Correct (Excludes X & S)
SECTION 3: SICK CHILD – DIARRHEA																							
NEXT QUESTIONS FOR CHILDREN 0–11 MONTHS ONLY																							
1	1	Child 0-11 months has had diarrhea in the last 2 weeks	YES																					
2	1 Alt	Child to be assessed for adequate treatment	if Q1 =YES write 1 if Q1 =NO write S																					
FOR THESE NEXT QUESTIONS -- ASSESS ONLY IF 1 Alt =1 -- if 1 Alt = S THEN DO NOT ASSESS AND MARK "S" IN ALL SPACES																							
3	3	What did you give [NAME] to treat the diarrhea? [IF Q2 = 2 or 88 THEN RECORD 0 IN THE SPACE]	1 or 2 or 3 (Acceptable options)																					
4	4	When (NAME) had diarrhea, was the quantity of liquids (and breastfeeding) that you gave her/him the same, more or less than normal?	MORE																					
5	5A	When (NAME) had diarrhea, was the quantity of food that you gave her/him the same, more or less than normal?	SAME or MORE (or EBF)																					
6	5B	When (NAME) was recuperating from diarrhea, was the quantity of food that you gave her/him the same, more or less than normal?	MORE (or EBF)																					
7	6	Where did you go first for treatment of (NAME)'s diarrhea?	Any acceptable options. Example: 1, 2, 3, 4																					

		NEXT QUESTIONS FOR CHILDREN 12–23 MONTHS ONLY																
8	1	Child 12–23 months has had diarrhea in the last 2 weeks	YES															
9	1 Alt	Child to be assessed for adequate treatment	if Q1 =YES write 1 if Q1 =NO write S															
		FOR THESE NEXT QUESTIONS -- ASSESS ONLY IF 1 Alt =1 – if 1 Alt = S THEN DO NOT ASSESS AND MARK "S" IN ALL SPACES																
10	3	What did you give [NAME] to treat the diarrhea? [IF Q2 = 2 or 88 THEN RECORD 0 IN THE SPACE]	(Acceptable Treatments)															
11	4A	When (NAME) had diarrhea, was the quantity of liquids (and breastfeeding) that you gave her/him the same, more or less than normal?	MORE															
12	5A	When (NAME) had diarrhea, was the quantity of food that you gave her/him the same, more or less than normal?	SAME or MORE (or EBF)															
13	5B	When (NAME) was recuperating from diarrhea, was the quantity of food that you gave her/him the same, more or less than normal?	MORE (or EBF)															
14	6B	Where did you go first for treatment of (NAME)'s diarrhea?	Any acceptable treatment. Example: 1, 2, 3, 4															
		SUMMARY OF DIARRHEA RESULTS: For all the following questions use the results of both Children 0-11 and Children 12–2 months3																
15		Total Children 0–23 months Sampled in Municipality	Count all of the entries with "1" or "0" in Table No. 1 and enter that number here =											+	Count all of the entries with "1" or "0" in Table No. 8 and enter that number here =			
16		Total Children 0–23 months with diarrhea in Municipality	Count all of the entries with "1" in Table No. 2 and enter that number here =											+	Count all of the entries with "1" in Table No. 9 and enter that number here =			
17		What did you give [NAME] to treat the diarrhea? [IF 2A = 2 or 88 THEN RECORD 0 IN THE SPACE]	Count all of the entries with "1" in Table No. 3 and enter that number here =											+	Count all of the entries with "1" in Table No. 10 and enter that number here =			
18		When (NAME) had diarrhea, was the quantity of liquids (and breastfeeding) that you gave her/him the same, more or less than normal?	Count all of the entries with "1" in Table No. 4 and enter that number here =											+	Count all of the entries with "1" in Table No. 11 and enter that number here =			
19		When (NAME) had diarrhea, was the quantity of food that you gave her/him the same, more or less than normal?	Count all of the entries with "1" in Table No. 5 and enter that number here =											+	Count all of the entries with "1" in Table No. 12 and enter that number here =			
20		When (NAME) was recuperating from diarrhea, was the quantity of food that you gave her/him the same, more or less than normal?	Count all of the entries with "1" in Table No. 6 and enter that number here =											+	Count all of the entries with "1" in Table No. 13 and enter that number here =			
21		Where did you go first for treatment of (NAME)'s diarrhea?	Count all of the entries with "1" in Table No. 7 and enter that number here =											+	Count all of the entries with "1" in Table No. 14 and enter that number here =			

SUMMARY TABLE FOR A MUNICIPALITY: Kwa-Zulu Natal, South Africa February 2002

Summary Tables: Exclusive Breastfeeding—Mothers of Children 0–11 Months

Municipality #1:   Municipality #2:   Municipality #3:   Municipality #4:   Municipality #5:

NO.	INDICATOR	Number Correct (or 1s) in Each Municipality (SA)/ Decision Rule (CIRCLE THE INDICATORS IN SAs BELOW STANDARD)					Total Number Correct (or 1s)	Total in Municipality or SA Sample (Exclude "Xs" and "Ss")					Total Catchment Area Sample	AVERAGE COVERAGE = Total Correct/ Total Sample Size	Target For this Assessment	BASELINE RESULT
		1	2	3	4	5		1	2	3	4	5				

SECTION 2: EXCLUSIVE BREASTFEEDING

If the Child is 0–5 months mark a "1".
If Child is 6–11 months mark an "S".

Next Question for Children 0–5 months ONLY -- The total in the sample size for this age group should equal the total in the above row.

Exclusive Breastfeeding

EXCLUSIVE BREASTFEEDING PREVALENCE = Total Exclusive Breastfeeding/Total Children 0–5 Months in Catchment Area Sample =

A-32   Appendix 7: Example Tabulation Tables for Sub-Samples

SUMMARY TABLE FOR A MUNICIPALITY: Kwa-Zulu Natal, South Africa February 2002
Treatment of the Sick Child --- Mothers of Children 0-23 Months

Municipality #1:		Municipality #2:					Municipality #3:	Municipality #4:						Municipality #5:		
Table No.	NO.	INDICATOR	Number Correct (or 1s) in Each Municipality (SA)/Decision Rule (CIRCLE THE INDICATORS IN SAs BELOW STANDARD)					Total Number Correct (or 1s)	Total in Municipality or SA Sample (Exclude "Xs" and "Ss")					Total Catchment Area Sample	AVERAGE COVERAGE = Total Correct / Total Sample Size	Target For this Assessment	BASELINE RESULT
			1	2	3	4	5		1	2	3	4	5				

SECTION 3: SICK CHILD -- DIARRHEA

SUMMARY OF DIARRHEA RESULTS: For all the following questions use the results of both Children 0–11 months and Children 12–23 months

1	1	Child 0-23 months sampled to assess diarrhea (line 15)															
2	1 Alt	Child 0-23 months with diarrhea to be assessed for adequate treatment (line 16)															
3		DIARRHEA PREVALENCE = Total Children with Diarrhea in Catchment Area (see Table No. 2) / Total Catchment Area Sample Size (See Table NO. 1)															
		FOR THE NEXT QUESTIONS INCLUDE IN THE DENOMINATOR ONLY THOSE CHILDREN WHO HAD DIARRHEA IN THE LAST TWO WEEKS AND ARE BEING ASSESSED FOR ADEQUATE TREATMENT															
4	---	What did you give [NAME] to treat the diarrhea?															
5	---	When (NAME) had diarrhea, was the quantity of liquids (and breastfeeding) that you gave her/him the same, more or less than normal?															
6	---	When (NAME) had diarrhea, was the quantity of food that you gave her/him the same, more or less than normal?															
7	---	When (NAME) was recuperating from diarrhea, was the quantity of food that you gave her/him the same, more or less than normal?															
8	---	Where did you go first for treatment of (NAME)'s diarrhea?															